*W*ellness
Nursing Diagnosis for
Health Promotion

~

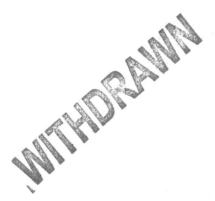

*W*ellness *Nursing Diagnosis for Health Promotion*

~

Karen M. Stolte, R.N., Ph.D.

Professor
University of Oklahoma College of Nursing
Oklahoma City, Oklahoma

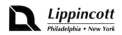

Lippincott
Philadelphia • New York

Acquisitions Editor: Mary P. Gyetvan, RN, MSN
Coordinating Editorial Assistant: Susan M. Keneally
Production Editor: Molly Dickmeyer

Library of Congress Cataloging-in-Publication Data
Stolte, Karen M.
     Wellness nursing diagnosis for health promotion / Karen M. Stolte.
        p.   cm.
     Includes bibliographical references and index.
     ISBN 0-397-55082-0 (alk. paper)
     1. Nursing diagnosis. 2. Health promotion. I. Title.
     [DNLM]: 1. Nursing Diagnosis. 2. Health Promotion. WY 100.4
     S876w 1996]
     RT48.6.S76   1996   RT
     610.73—dc20   48.6
     DNLM/DLC   .S76   95-38990
     for Library of Congress   CIP
                                1996

     The material contained in this volume was submitted as previously unpublished material, except in the instances in which credit has been given to the source from which some of the illustrative material was derived.
     Any procedure or practice described in this book should be applied by the healthcare practitioner under appropriate supervision in accordance with professional standards of care used with regard to the unique circumstances that apply in each practice situation. Care has been taken to confirm the accuracy of information presented and to describe generally accepted practices. However, the authors, editors, and publisher cannot accept any responsibility for errors or omissions or for any consequences from application of the information in this book and make no warranty, express or implied, with respect to the contents of the book.
     The authors and publisher have exerted every effort to ensure that drug selection and dosage set forth in this text are in accordance with current recommendations and practice at the time of publication. However, in view of ongoing research, changes in government regulations, and the constant flow of information relating to drug therapy and drug reactions, the reader is urged to check the package insert for each drug for any change in indications and dosage and for added warnings and precautions. This is particularly important when the recommended agent is a new or infrequently employed drug.
     Materials appearing in this book prepared by individuals as part of their official duties as U.S. Government employees are not covered by the above-mentioned copyright.

     9   8   7   6   5   4   3   2   1

CONTRIBUTORS

Dorothy C. Belknap, R.N., Ph.D.
Associate Professor
University of Oklahoma College of Nursing
Oklahoma City, Oklahoma
(Chapter 12)

Lynda J. Davidson, R.N., Ph.D.
Assistant Professor
University of Pittsburgh School of Nursing
Pittsburgh, Pennsylvania
(Chapter 12)

REVIEWERS

Linda Anderson, RN, MA
Nursing Faculty
Central Lakes Community College
Brainerd, Minnesota

Connie S. Austin, RN, MAEd, MSN
Associate Professor of Nursing
Azusa Pacific University
Azusa, California

Lou Ann Boose, RN, MSN
Assistant Professor of Nursing
Harrisburg Area Community College
Harrisburg, Pennsylvania

Cynthia S. Roberts, RN, MSN
Faculty Instructor, Nursing Program
University of Southern Indiana
Evansville, Indiana

Preface

This book is based on the belief that the time has come for wellness nursing diagnoses. The use of wellness nursing diagnoses complements problem-oriented nursing diagnoses to provide a holistic approach to client care. Not only can wellness nursing diagnoses improve the health status of the well client, but they can provide hope for the ill client by incorporating positive aspects of life and health into nursing care. The enthusiasm that students have shown for wellness nursing diagnoses is overwhelming. Students from all clinical areas verbalize amazement at how positively clients respond to discussion of their strengths. The positive response of practicing nurses to this approach further confirms the value of wellness nursing diagnoses.

PURPOSE OF THE BOOK

The purpose of this book is to provide a foundation for students and practicing nurses that: (1) defines the concept of wellness nursing diagnosis and reviews literature on the topic, (2) describes the usefulness of wellness nursing diagnoses, and (3) presents one framework for writing such a diagnosis. Most wellness nursing diagnoses in this book reflect a process approach. Some reflect patterns of patient behaviors rather than specific processes. Others indicate that the client has completed the process and needs continued reinforcement of these new behaviors. However, any of these diagnoses are appropriate to use with clients. Finally, the book presents a beginning taxonomy of wellness nursing diagnoses, a springboard for the development of future generations of diagnoses which could, in turn, be validated using client data. The reader is encouraged to develop additional wellness diagnoses.

STRUCTURE OF THE BOOK

This book is divided into 5 units. Unit 1 discusses the nature of wellness nursing diagnoses. Unit II reviews wellness nursing diagnoses across the lifespan. Unit III presents wellness nursing diagnoses in special health care environments. Unit IV extends the concept of wellness nursing diagnoses to groups. Unit V reviews wellness nursing diagnosis literature.

Initial chapters explore the increased interest in health and wellness in our society, as well as the wellness nursing diagnosis controversy. One chapter describes how to write a wellness nursing diagnosis. The recommended format used in this book includes a client response (first portion of the diagnosis) and related factors (second portion of the diagnosis) identified as a condition. Because conditions arise from client data, lists of conditions have not been provided, but examples are included in chapter discussions. Another early chapter shows how to assess and build on client strengths.

Remaining chapters are organized in a consistent manner. They describe the kinds of healthy processes specific to the chapter topic. Assessment questions and sample wellness diagnoses are provided for each topic. A case study in each of these chapters helps the reader apply theory to clinical practice. Chapters conclude with detailed tables highlighting the relationship between wellness nursing diagnoses, client or group behaviors, and nursing interventions.

A detailed review of the literature is provided, and a separate appendix lists wellness nursing diagnoses by chapter for easy retrieval.

Acknowledgments

A book such as this could not be written without the help and support of others. Faculty who have reviewed chapters and provided valuable insight include Drs. Mary Allen, Constance Baker, Herbert Nishikawa, Carol Mannahan, Sheila Myers, Ruth Seideman, and Teresa Smiley. Informal support from Drs. Andrea Bircher and June Schmele also has been greatly appreciated. The chapter by Dr. Dorothy Belknap and Dr. Lynda Davidson on use of wellness nursing diagnoses in critical care gives an exciting flavor to the book. I sincerely thank them for their input. The graduate students who allowed me to modify their case studies for inclusion in the book include Ms. Marjorie Pyrom, Ms. Glenda Bell, and Ms. Kay Farrell. Ms. Pamela Props and Ms. Marian Schumacher were helpful in examining the usefulness of wellness nursing diagnoses in home health care. Lastly, my parents, Lucille and Fariss, have always provided support for my endeavors. For that encouragement and love, I am extremely grateful.

Contents

UNIT II
Wellness Nursing Diagnosis Across the Lifespan

UNIT III
Wellness Nursing Diagnosis in Special/Selected Health Care Environments

UNIT IV
Wellness Nursing Diagnosis for
Groups and Aggregates

UNIT V
Wellness Nursing Diagnosis in Literature

Unit **I**

~

*T*he Nature of Wellness Nursing Diagnosis

~

1
~

Wellness in Nursing Care and Nursing Diagnosis

Historically, most nursing and health care activities have dealt with treatment of disease or responses to disease. Although community health nurses have worked with clients in areas of health promotion for a number of years, access to these clients has been through referrals focusing on illness, tertiary care, or prevention of further disease. In general, health promotion has received minimal attention.

During the last decade, interest in health promotion and wellness has soared in the United States. Articles related to fitness or development of healthy lifestyles are found in lay magazines, videotapes on physical fitness abound, and the professional literature contains articles describing wellness, health, or freedom from illness.

Health has been defined as "a dynamic state of being in which the developmental and behavioral potential of an individual is realized to the fullest extent possible" (American Nurses Association, *Social Policy Statement*, 1980, p. 5). The U.S. government publication *Healthy People 2000* (1990) and the PEW report *Healthy America: Practitioners for 2005* (1991) emphasize goals of health promotion and disease prevention. If practitioners for the future are to be competent in the areas of primary and secondary prevention and are to encourage healthy lifestyles, a focus on wellness is needed.

Dever (1991) asserts that problems in lifestyle, environment, and human biology account for a much higher percentage of deaths than inadequacies in the health care system. Believing that present national health policies do not provide methods that effectively reduce mortality and morbidity, Dever proposes a holistic wellness policy and emphasizes the need for a public policy where health care professionals are advocates in promoting health. Such a policy would include the areas of health enhancement, interaction between environment and health status (both individual and community), and the health care system.

The escalating cost of health care also necessitates a shift from treatment of illness to disease prevention and health promotion. Historically, insurance coverage has been for treatment of disease rather than for prevention of illness. The cost of hospitalization in critical care units as well as the cost of diagnostic technology is often prohibitive for the consumer. In addition, a major illness can exhaust a family's resources, both financial and emotional, regardless of insurance coverage.

If illness can be prevented, health care costs can be reduced. The cost of health maintenance is far less than the cost of treatment of disease. In addition, health care resources are limited. If the focus were on health promotion and disease prevention, these resources could be used more effectively for a larger number of people. Health maintenance organizations and wellness centers are examples of organizations that emphasize health promotion as a way to reallocate and conserve resources.

～ *Definition of Wellness*

Health is not merely the absence of disease. The wellness literature is prolific with definitions of wellness and health. Kulbok and Baldwin (1992) note that conceptual confusion exists among the many terms used to describe health promotion behaviors. They assert that a paradigm shift has not yet taken place, since health promotion behaviors are used merely to achieve the goal of disease prevention rather than high-level wellness and self-actualization.

Commonalities exist among the definitions of health and wellness. First, wellness is described as a *process* that is continually evolving to higher and higher levels of functioning. Such evolution implies change and growth as well as a balance of energies that preserve system integrity. Patterns of behavior that foster the client's potential for this higher level of functioning must be identified and strengthened.

The client is an *active* participant in achieving this wellness state. Goals of self-actualization, personal fulfillment, and increased well-being reinforce the notion that the client assumes a personal responsibility for health. To enhance fulfillment of these goals, the nurse seeks to empower the client in the quest for goal attainment. In essence, the nurse and the client share accountability for the client's wellness state.

Various types of lifestyle modifications that will lead to higher levels of functioning are presented in the wellness literature. Nutrition, physical exercise, and stress reduction are often mentioned for consideration when planning alterations in lifestyle. A lifestyle that promotes health includes self-directed actions that enhance or maintain wellness and self-actualization or self-fulfillment. Developing and sustaining that lifestyle requires motivation, goal setting, purposeful action, and positive reinforcement.

～ *Nursing and Wellness*

Where does the nurse fit in wellness care? Clients need to be helped to understand their strengths and weaknesses as well as to find ways to function at the best possible level. Nursing care can facilitate this understanding. Poland (1992) describes three mechanisms intrinsic to health promotion: self-care, mutual aid (social support), and promotion of healthy environments.

Identification of areas where the client can give self-care, assessment of social support networks, and assessment of the environment in which the client lives and interacts are the first steps in providing nursing care that will help the client achieve wellness. After such assessment has occurred, interventions that facilitate the client's goal attainment need to be implemented. These interventions could focus on enhancing the client's ability to give self-care, helping the client develop a social support system, or maintaining or altering the environment to facilitate wellness efforts (see Table 1.1).

Ability to give self-care can be enhanced by gaining knowledge about health and wellness and acquiring the skills, such as stress management techniques, needed to achieve specific wellness goals. The nurse can help the client identify sources of social support. In addition, mutual exploration of ways to develop a support system can be effective in helping the client obtain social support. In like fashion, the nurse and client can discuss ways to alter the environment that will increase opportunities to practice wellness behaviors.

The current emphasis on cost containment limits the amount of time nurses have to work with clients. Therefore, strategies need to be developed that help clients interact in a positive way with their home environment since they will not

Table 1.1. Nursing Aspects of Wellness Promotion

Areas of Assessment →	*Mutual Nurse–Client Goal Setting* →	*Interventions for Wellness*
Strengths in self-care ability, skills, knowledge, role attainment, accomplishment of developmental tasks		Reinforce or enhance self-care ability, skills, knowledge, role attainment, accomplishment of developmental tasks
Social support networks		Strengthen social support
Client's environment		Maintain or alter the environment

be in a health care setting very long (Montgomery and Webster, 1993). One strategy is a health focus rather than a problem focus where nursing interventions are based on client strengths. These strengths are used to help clients deal with health care issues.

Assessing a combination of client strengths, concerns, lifestyle patterns, and skills provides the nurse with a foundation upon which to build a wide variety of interventions. This broad approach to care enables the client to look for future possibilities and make changes that will lead to good health.

Although the client who is not ill may be able to reach wellness goals without help, support from a nurse can often enhance the client's coping efforts and reduce the time needed to reach these goals. Health promotion and wellness can also be achieved by clients who have some degree of illness. Regardless of type of illness or disability, a wellness focus urges the client to strive for the highest possible level of wellness.

~ *Nursing and Wellness Diagnoses*

The increasing emphasis on health and wellness in our society makes consideration of wellness nursing diagnoses an imperative for the profession. Although the place of wellness nursing diagnoses in caring for healthy clients seems obvious, support of healthy behaviors and healthy lifestyles will also help clients who are ill cope with their illness and its effects by providing them with a reference that draws attention to past and present strengths. This recognition of strengths can decrease vulnerability in the present illness.

In addition, a complementary approach using both wellness and problem-oriented diagnoses for the ill client fosters a holistic approach to care. Rather than focusing on only one aspect of life, i.e., illness, the nurse values client strengths and uses them to help achieve client goals of improved health.

Wellness nursing diagnoses can be used in a wide variety of ambulatory care settings where clients seek information about health and illness. They can be implemented in acute care settings where clients present a wide variety of behaviors—some related to illness and others related to health. In addition, wellness centers that focus on health promotion present an ideal setting for wellness nursing diagnoses. Recognition of diagnoses for healthy clients encourages the use of nursing diagnoses in these settings and helps clarify the nurse's role.

When formulating nursing diagnoses, the literature emphasizes the need for problem identification. However, over the years, a small but tenacious group of nurses has provided rationale for the use of wellness nursing diagnoses (Martens, 1986; Lee and Frenn, 1987; Popkess-Vawter, 1991; Stolte, 1994). Warren (1991) proposes that several axes be developed within the North American Nursing Diagnosis Association (NANDA) nursing diagnosis taxonomy to facilitate delineation of diagnoses for specific ages, types of clients (individuals, family, community), and illness and wellness states.

Currently, the majority of approved NANDA nursing diagnoses are problem oriented. They usually deal with illness or unhealthy responses or, in the case of risk diagnoses, focus on the vulnerable individual, family, or community. Since NANDA revised the definition of nursing diagnosis at the ninth conference to include "life processes" as well as "actual or potential health problems" (Carpenito, 1991, p. 65), greater latitude for consideration of wellness diagnoses now exists. However, of the approximately 130 nursing diagnoses listed by NANDA (1994), only 8 reflect healthy responses or potential for healthy responses.

～ Definition of Wellness Nursing Diagnosis

How are wellness diagnoses defined in the literature? NANDA (1994) states that wellness nursing diagnoses "describe human responses to levels of wellness in an individual, family, or community that have a potential for enhancement to a higher state" (p. 102).

Carpenito (1995) asserts that wellness diagnoses are one-part statements that include a label only. Because the client desires a higher level of functioning, there is no need to identify contributing factors. In cases where the client is functioning adequately and no effort is made toward improvement, Carpenito maintains that positive functioning assessment statements would be included in the assessment data, but a wellness diagnosis would not be formulated as a guide for action.

Essentially, Carpenito proposes that a wellness diagnosis be used only in cases where the focus is on improved functioning and the goal is progression from one level of wellness to a higher level of wellness. She describes two cues that indicate justification for a wellness nursing diagnosis: "(1) desire for higher level of wellness and (2) effective present status or function" (p. 17). Yet some conceptual confusion exists when she presents a wellness nursing diagnosis related to a negative factor: *"health-seeking behaviors related to insufficient knowledge of new parent role"* (p. 19). If the emphasis is on client strengths, then the related factors should reveal a strength also. Otherwise, the emphasis is still on negative behaviors or deficits. An alternative diagnosis would be *health-seeking behaviors related to anticipated role change*.

Stolte (1994) refers to a wellness nursing diagnosis as a "conclusion from assessment data which focuses on patterns of wellness, healthy responses, or client strengths" (p. 145). This conclusion results from the integration of client data and the nurse's knowledge base, allowing the nurse to make a clinical judgment resulting in a nursing diagnosis.

Stolte suggests a process approach to wellness diagnosis that focuses on progressive attainment of health behaviors or completion of developmental tasks. Underlying this process approach is the proposition that the nurse facilitates healthy processes in order to attain health-oriented goals. This approach to wellness diagnoses includes those situations where the nurse helps the client complete developmental transitions, achieve higher levels of wellness, or attain wellness states. It also gives recognition and credibility to the place of nursing in those situations.

Because these wellness diagnoses are used to identify strengths as well as provide a foundation for interventions that help the client complete the healthy processes occurring in his or her life, they may contain one or two parts. In those instances, where a contributing factor can be identified, it is included because such contributing factors maintain or enhance the healthy process. Therefore, nursing action is directed toward enhancing the contributing condition as well as helping the client progress through the process.

Most authors do not differentiate between positive functioning statements and wellness nursing diagnoses and propose that wellness nursing diagnoses be used in all healthy situations. Various terms such as *positive nursing diagnosis, wellness diagnosis,* and *health-oriented diagnosis* are used interchangeably in the literature. In the past, approaches to wellness nursing diagnoses have ranged widely from Pender's (1989) proposal for two taxonomies of nursing diagnoses (one for potential/actual health/illness problems and one for strengths and resources) to a manual of wellness diagnoses based on functional health patterns written by Houldin, Saltstein, and Ganley (1987). Some authors discuss wellness diagnoses exclusively whereas others focus on problem-oriented diagnoses and include one or two wellness diagnoses.

∼ *The Wellness Nursing Diagnosis Controversy*

Although many nurses have expressed an interest in wellness nursing diagnoses, a debate still exists about whether or not such diagnoses are appropriate for nursing (see Table 1.2). Arguments against wellness nursing diagnoses are centered around three issues:

- Acute care settings focus on actual or potential problems; using wellness nursing diagnoses places an additional burden on resources that are currently pushed to the limit.
- Clients who do not have problems do not need nursing care.
- Little reimbursement is currently available for wellness care.

The following paragraphs are a rebuttal to these arguments. Table 1.2 provides a summary of arguments for and against wellness nursing diagnoses.

Acute Care Settings

A combination of wellness-oriented and problem-oriented nursing diagnoses is useful when the client has an acute or chronic illness. In general, acutely ill clients bring many strengths and

Table 1.2. The Wellness Nursing Diagnosis Controversy

Arguments Against	Arguments For
Acute care settings have a problem focus and a heavy workload	Wellness diagnoses complement problem-oriented diagnoses and provide holistic assessment. Other client advantages: 1. Focus on past and present strengths 2. Provide evidence of past and present coping ability
The client who has no problems does not need a nurse	Nurses facilitate progression through normal developmental and maturational tasks even if no problem exists. A health-oriented focus provides encouragement that success is possible.
Payment is not available for wellness care	Cost-containment efforts for wellness care are becoming directed toward health. Wellness diagnoses help build a case for the nurse's role in the wellness arena.

past experiences to bear upon their ability to cope with a current illness. In fact, clients have more healthy responses than unhealthy ones. Some experts believe that no problem should be recorded without describing a concomitant strength.

Identification and reinforcement of strengths decreases vulnerability, provides evidence of past coping ability, and encourages recognition that the client can handle the present situation. Thus, these strengths are not only part of the diagnosis, but the nurse actively intervenes to facilitate further development and use of these abilities. Pray (1992) emphasizes this need to focus on an individual's competence and ability in order to incorporate the uniqueness of the individual into the treatment plan.

Although the wellness nursing diagnosis may not have first priority when selecting diagnoses for planning of care during acute illness, inclusion of this type of diagnosis does help provide a holistic assessment of the client. In client situations where the illness is chronic, wellness diagnoses encourage success rather than failure and may help the client cope with the problems of living with chronic illness. Recognizing and nurturing client strengths can also help a client die with dignity in those instances where recovery is not possible.

Client with No Problems

The belief that a client who has no problems does not need a nurse eliminates goals that deal with the normal response to developmental or maturational events in a client's life. This belief also presumes there is no place for a nurse in wellness centers. Should we discontinue much of the health teaching and health supervision done in maternity and community health nursing just because problems do not exist at the moment?

An important function of wellness diagnoses is to focus on the developmental/maturational tasks that need to be accomplished during various life transitions. Clients may complete these tasks without nursing intervention. However, in our mobile society, some clients lack social support, have high stress levels, and possess limited resources. By providing social support and other resources, such as knowledge and skill, the nurse can facilitate the client's efforts to complete these tasks. As a result, they may be achieved more quickly and/or with less stress than if the client worked alone.

In an attempt to find a place for nursing actions with clients where no emergent problems have been identified, the label of "potential problems" has emerged. The label may be appropriate in certain situations where a potential for infection or a potential for skin breakdown is clearly a possibility. Unfortunately, the term is frequently overused in nursing practice, especially with healthy clients. To build a case for health teaching by examining potential problems seems to be contradictory because the data do not necessarily provide evidence for a problem orientation. If there are data to support the possibility of a potential problem, the label can be used. However, if one is not careful, a minor problem can be blown out of proportion in order to justify nursing care.

Similarly, NANDA (1994) uses the term "risk nursing diagnosis" to identify clients who are vulnerable and at risk for problems even though no such problem currently exists. Risk factors are identified and actions are directed toward reducing the risk. Although some nurses maintain that risk diagnoses are useful for health promotion, the same problems emerge as with "potential problem." Emphasis remains on problem areas or weaknesses (vulnerabilities) rather than on existing or potential strengths.

Identification of potential problems or risks can lead clients to question their ability as well as create feelings that negative outcomes are inevitable. Thus, normal processes may be impeded because the client may become discouraged and think these processes are not achievable. Self-fulfilling prophecies may occur if the client lives up to the label of a potential problem.

For example, a diagnosis of *potential problem in maternal role attainment* can create a negative set, cause the client to question her ability to carry out the mothering role, and deter her efforts toward healthy mothering behaviors. In contrast, a well-ness nursing diagnosis of *progressive attainment of maternal role* is much more encouraging for both the patient and the nurse.

Payment for Wellness Care

Currently, little third-party payment is available for health prevention. As health care policy is revised in this country, it seems inevitable that a greater emphasis on health promotion and disease prevention will occur. The importance of cutting health care costs makes it necessary to provide a rationale for all care. Effective ways to communicate the cost of that care are also needed if one is to be reimbursed.

Because nursing diagnoses guide and direct nursing care, they form a foundation for goal development, which in turn pro-vides a basis for interventions that can be used to facilitate goal achievement. Development of wellness nursing diagnoses and goals that focus on healthy client outcomes, achieved through nursing intervention, is the first step toward creating a proposal that demonstrates the role of the nurse in wellness care and pro-vides a rationale for reimbursement for cost-effective care.

Communication and Professional Development

Other purposes for the use of wellness nursing diagnoses are described in the literature. One purpose is to communicate client strengths to other health care professionals. In this instance, client strengths or healthy responses are assessed and reported, but are not considered in other parts of the nursing process. However, using wellness diagnoses for communication only is a limited view of their use.

A final argument for the use of wellness nursing diagnoses is that use of nursing diagnosis as a foundation for nursing care advances the profession. Nurses who work with healthy clients such as pregnant women or who work in wellness set-tings have had difficulty applying problem-oriented nursing diagnoses in their clinical areas. Therefore, they have not used nursing diagnoses in practice. The availability of wellness nursing diagnoses will increase their efforts to use nursing diagnoses. This availability will also enhance the use of a common language in nursing, facilitate communication among health care professionals, and build a professional base for nursing.

SUMMARY

Although controversy still exists about the usefulness of wellness nursing diagnoses, interest in this topic is increasing. Consideration of the effectiveness of wellness nursing diagnoses reveals that they are useful in helping the ill client recognize strengths in spite of illness, in clarifying the role of the nurse with healthy clients, and in paving the way for third-party reimbursement for wellness care.

Because a nursing diagnosis facilitates goal development and guides patient care, identification of healthy responses for wellness nursing diagnoses provides a shift from the negative to the positive. Healthy responses are often part of a process that can be facilitated or encouraged by the nurse. Learning new skills, attaining a new role, or working toward a specific goal also involves normal processes that take variable amounts of time and effort in order to achieve mastery of the skill, consistent role performance, or goal attainment.

Rather than identifying potential problems or expecting clients to accomplish new learning in an unrealistic time frame (a function of short hospital stays), client efforts toward accomplishment of healthy processes need to be enhanced and reinforced. The use of wellness diagnoses is the first step in this paradigm shift that recognizes wellness states are not static and the presence of a problem is not a prerequisite for nursing care.

References

Carpenito, L.J. (1991). The NANDA definition of nursing diagnosis. In R.M. Carroll-Johnson (ed.), *Classification of Nursing Diagnoses: Proceedings of the Ninth Conference North American Nursing Diagnosis Association* (pp. 65–71). Philadelphia: Lippincott.

Carpenito, L.J. (1995). *Nursing Diagnosis: Application to Clinical Practice.* Philadelphia: Lippincott.

Dever, G.E.A. (1991). *Community Health Analysis: Global Awareness at the Local Level* (2nd ed). Gaithersburg: Aspen.

Healthy People 2000: National Health Promotion and Disease Prevention Objectives (1990). Washington, DC: United States Department of Health and Human Services, USPHS.

Houldin, A.D., Saltstein, S.W., and Ganley, K.M. (1987). *Nursing Diagnoses for Wellness.* Philadelphia: Lippincott.

Kulbok, P.A., and Baldwin, J.H. (1992). From preventive health behavior to health promotion: Advancing a positive construct of health. *Advances in Nursing Science, 14*(4), 50–64.

Lee, H.A., and Frenn, M.D. (1987). The use of nursing diagnoses for health promotion in community practice. *Nursing Clinics of North America, 22,* 981–987.

Martens, K. (1986). Let's diagnose strengths, not just problems. *American Journal of Nursing, 86,* 192–193.

Montgomery, C., and Webster, D.C. (1993). Caring and nursing's metaparadigm: Can they survive the era of managed care? *Perspectives in Psychiatric Care, 29*(4), 5–12.

Nursing Diagnoses: Definitions and Classifications 1995–1996 (1994). Philadelphia: North American Nursing Diagnosis Association.

Pender, N.J. (1989). Languaging a health perspective for NANDA taxonomy on research and theory. In R.M. Carroll-Johnson (ed.), *Proceedings of the Eighth Conference North American Nursing Diagnosis Association* (pp. 31–36). Philadelphia: Lippincott.

Poland, B.D. (1992). Learning to "walk our talk": The implications of sociological theory for research methodologies in health promotion. *Canadian Journal of Public Health,* supplement 1, S31–S36.

Popkess-Vawter, S. (1991). Wellness nursing diagnoses: To be or not to be? *Nursing Diagnosis, 2*(1), 20–25.

Pray, J.E. (1992). Maximizing the patient's uniqueness and strengths: A challenge for home health care. *Social Work in Health Care, 17*(3), 71–79.

Social Policy Statement (1980). Kansas City: American Nurses Association.

Stolte, K. (1994). Health-oriented nursing diagnoses: Development and use. In R.M. Carroll-Johnson and M. Paquette (eds.), *Classification of Nursing Diagnoses: Proceedings of the 10th Conference*

North American Nursing Diagnosis Association (pp. 143–148). Philadelphia: Lippincott.

Sugars, D.A., O'Neil, E.H., and Bader, J.D. (eds.) (1991). *Healthy America: Practitioners for 2005, an Agenda for Action for U.S. Health Professional Schools.* Durham, NC: The Pew Health Professions Commission.

Warren, J.J. (1991). Implications for introducing axes into a classification system. In R.M. Carroll-Johnson (ed.), *Classification of Nursing Diagnoses: Proceedings of the Ninth Conference North American Nursing Diagnosis Association* (pp. 38–43). Philadelphia: Lippincott.

2
~

Developing a Wellness Nursing Diagnosis

Chapter 1 included pros and cons for wellness nursing diagnoses. In addition to these theoretical issues, nurses who have had experience in writing wellness nursing diagnoses have consistently remarked that such diagnoses are exactly what is needed to reflect their client data. Others have stated that wellness diagnoses are exciting and challenging to write and provide encouragement for clients. The idea of working on something that is positive rather than focusing on illness or negative behaviors generates enthusiasm among nurses, nursing students, and clients. The purpose of this chapter is to provide the reader with a guide for writing wellness nursing diagnoses.

The procedure for data collection to support a wellness diagnosis is the same as that for support of a problem-oriented diagnosis. Assessment of client strengths through client interview, discussion with family members, or review of the client's chart provides data that the nurse analyzes for patterns of health-related behavior, or clusters of healthy characteristics. An identified client strength does not automatically become a response for inclusion in a nursing diagnosis. The nurse arrives at a wellness nursing diagnosis by combining client behaviors that are seen in the clinical situation with theoretical knowledge about wellness, health, transitional events, and normal growth and development. Writing a wellness diagnosis will be easier if the nurse considers what kind of health-related processes a client may be undergoing.

~ *Health-Related Processes*

Looking at client behaviors in terms of completing a process facilitates the nurse's development of wellness diagnoses. A process is involved if the client must complete several steps or phases before the final goal is reached. For example, one can describe behaviors that indicate the early stages of maternal attachment, or behaviors that demonstrate the first steps of assuming a role, but different behaviors are involved in later parts of these processes. Therefore, by identifying these behaviors and the steps involved, the nurse can determine the client's progress in completion of the process and use that information to formulate the response portion of the wellness diagnosis.

Some processes where wellness nursing diagnoses might be used include the following:

- Gaining new information
- Wound healing
- Learning new skills
- Improving physical functional status
- Weaning from ventilators
- Acquiring new roles
- Achieving maturational/developmental tasks
- Developing new strengths

Thinking about the sequential steps involved in physiological recovery, making changes in one's lifestyle, adapting to illness, and learning new information will help the nurse identify the progression through which the client must move in order to achieve the goal. If the client is in the early stages of this process, the response portion of the wellness nursing diagnosis can be written to indicate which of the initial steps describe the client situation; the goal becomes completion of the process and the nurse intervenes to facilitate goal attainment.

Learning, whether it involves assimilating new information or developing a new skill, begins with being able to identify the concepts that need to be learned and proceeds to analysis and synthesis before mastery occurs. Role acquisition is also a process as the individual takes on the role through observation, mimicry, and practice. As the role is practiced, role acquisition occurs, but may take several months. Developmental or maturational tasks are also achieved over time. As examples, some steps involved in several of these processes are presented in Table 2.1.

Although a client may not have completed a process, he or she may have accomplished part of it. Instead of considering partial success a potential problem, viewing that progress as realistic in light of time constraints or other factors leads to wellness nursing diagnoses.

Table 2.1. Examples of Steps of Health-Related Processes

Process	Process Steps
GAIN NEW KNOWLEDGE	Recall, identify, acquire information → Restate, reorder, put in own words → Apply information
LEARN NEW SKILL	Observation → Practice with supervision → Competence in skill → Proficiency in skill
ACQUIRE NEW ROLE	Observe role behaviors → Mimicry of behaviors → Acceptance or rejection of behaviors for own life → Incorporate behaviors into lifestyle

~ *Writing a Wellness Nursing Diagnosis*

One-Part Diagnoses

A modification of the Mundinger and Jauron (1975) framework for nursing diagnosis development is useful. Although this framework is old, the author's 20 years of experience in writing wellness diagnoses using this framework, and in teaching it to students, validates its worth.

Mundinger and Jauron define nursing diagnosis as a two-part statement composed of a client *response* to a contributing *condition*. Although they use unhealthy responses, substitution of healthy responses is possible. This definition is consistent with the NANDA components for a nursing diagnosis. Response can be considered similar to the diagnostic label in the NANDA format and condition is similar to etiology or related factors.

When writing a wellness nursing diagnosis, it is often difficult to identify a particular condition that contributes to the client response, especially if the strength has existed for some time. If conditions cannot be identified, a one-part diagnosis can be used, i.e., the response only. The wellness diagnoses in this book are client responses only. Because conditions vary with specific client situations and emerge from client data, no attempt to identify conditions has been made.

Writing the response section of the wellness diagnosis in a process format helps avoid confusion between a wellness diagnosis and a goal. The response portion of a wellness nursing diagnosis identifies where the client is in the process and assists in goal development.

Without this process approach, the response portion of the diagnosis often cannot be differentiated from the goal to be achieved or may lead other nurses to believe the goal has already been attained. For example, a response of *maternal–infant attachment* is ambiguous. The statement can mean any one of the following:

- It is the response portion of a wellness diagnosis.
- Attachment has already occurred and no further intervention is needed.
- The desired goal is maternal–infant attachment.

Since goals and interventions are based on the nursing diagnosis, confusion could arise and desired outcomes might not be achieved if the goal is not clear or if description of the client response is not accurate.

In contrast, a diagnosis with a response of *beginning maternal–infant attachment* indicates that the process of attachment is occurring and the potential for a mature relationship exists even though it has not yet been accomplished. The goal for this response would be maternal–infant attachment, and as interventions, the nurse could enable the mother to learn more about her infant by providing opportunities for interaction with the infant as well as describing infant capabilities and characteristics.

A process approach to nursing diagnosis implies that the nurse can facilitate client progression through the process. Identification of the condition that contributes to the client response allows the nurse to use interventions that reinforce this condition. Logically, if the condition is reinforced, the client response will also be reinforced and goal attainment will be enhanced.

A process approach clarifies the role of the nurse with clients who do not have an illness but need health supervision, health teaching, or assistance with developmental or maturational transitions. In addition, clients who are ill undergo many of the same processes when learning about their illness, adapting to chronic illness, or completing developmental tasks. Therefore, process diagnoses can be used with both healthy and ill clients.

Most, but not all, of the wellness nursing diagnoses presented in this book reflect a process approach. However, some do not. Several reasons exist for this inconsistency. Some strengths do not lend themselves to a process approach. In addition, the level of conceptualization varies widely among the diagnoses presented. Some reflect patterns of patient behaviors rather than specific processes. Others indicate that the client has completed the process, yet needs continued reinforcement of these behaviors. Still others indicate a strong process approach. Any of these diagnoses can be used with clients and may be refined with use. The first priority is to develop and use wellness diagnoses; the second is to use the process approach as much as possible.

Two-Part Diagnoses

If the nurse can identify specific conditions that contribute to the client response, it is ideal to include them in the diagnosis because they give direction to nursing care. In general, if a two-part diagnosis is used, the short-term goals relate to the condition and the long-term goals relate to the response (see Display 2.1).

DISPLAY 2.1

Relationship Among Assessment, Wellness Nursing Diagnoses, and Goals

Assessment		Wellness Diagnosis	
Observational data $\rightarrow$	*Healthy Response*	*related to a*	*Contributing Condition*
+	↓		↓
Nurse's Knowledge of Health-Related Processes	*Long-Term Goal*		*Short-Term Goal*

In wellness diagnoses, such conditions generally reinforce, amplify, or maintain the client's response. The nurse's efforts are directed at supporting or enhancing the condition, which then fosters or strengthens the client's response. In most cases, several conditions may have contributed to the client response. The nurse must decide which condition will be the focus of care. Generally, one condition will stand out in the client data.

For instance, if a client response is *beginning maternal attachment* (indicated by calling the infant by name and holding the infant in *en face* position), the nurse might determine that initiation of breastfeeding, early contact with the infant, or systematic playing with the fetus has reinforced this response. Of these three conditions, the one the nurse can influence the most is breastfeeding. Therefore, this condition would become part of the nursing diagnosis: *beginning maternal attachment related to initiation of breastfeeding.*

With a two-part diagnosis, short-term goals are usually related to the condition portion of the diagnosis. In the previous example about breastfeeding, the short-term goal could be: The client will have a successful breastfeeding experience as evidenced by (1) infant weight gain, (2) statements of satisfaction about breastfeeding, and (3) duration of breastfeeding of at least 4 weeks. Since successful breastfeeding will enhance maternal attachment, achievement of the short-term goals will, in turn, facilitate attainment of the long-term goal, which is maternal attachment.

～ *Relationship Between Goals and Diagnosis*

Before goals are determined, the nurse shares the diagnosis with the client to seek input or validation that it is an area where mutually acceptable goals can be developed for client care. Sharing these wellness diagnoses also helps the client see progress, which in turn will increase motivation to complete the process. Remembering that goals are conceptual statements of desirable behaviors, the client and the nurse work together to determine what is an acceptable, feasible, satisfying goal. This mutual goal setting increases the probability of achievement of desired outcomes. Without it, the nurse's goals may differ from those of the client, expectations may be unclear, and the probability of attaining the goal decreases.

Goals also include criteria, written in terms of specific behaviors or observable data, which make it possible to determine if they are met. If they are not met within the specified time frame, reassessment may reveal that goals need to be changed or refined, alternative interventions are required, or in some instances, reevaluation of the nursing diagnosis is necessary.

In the processes described earlier, goals relate to achievement of maturational/developmental tasks, retention of information, skill acquisition, role mastery, or maintaining or developing strengths, respectively. The nurse intervenes to facilitate task achievement, provide information, teach or reinforce new skills, foster role attainment, or enhance strengths.

Examples of QUALIFIERS a nurse might use when developing goals for the diagnoses presented in this book include the following

- Attainment
- Continued
- Increased
- Sustained
- Completion
- Acceptance

Other examples are given in Table 2.2.

~ Common Obstacles to Writing Wellness Diagnoses

Nurses are accustomed to identifying problems and using problem-oriented nursing diagnoses. Therefore, it is difficult to switch to identification of client strengths and development of wellness diagnoses. In fact, nurses often flounder when a problem cannot be identified because they are used to look-

Table 2.2. Suggested Wording of Goals for Healthy Responses

Healthy Response	*Long-Term Goal*
Beginning attainment of maternal role	**Attainment** of maternal role
Pride in ability to master new role	**Continued** pride in ability to master new role
Beginning ability to maintain stress reduction	**Increased** ability to maintain stress reduction
Satisfaction with past and present life as lived	**Sustained** satisfaction with past and present life as lived
Reevaluation of personal goals	**Revised** personal goals and/or expressed satisfaction with current goals
Beginning acceptance of self	**Acceptance** of self
Improving nutritional intake	**Adequate** nutritional intake
Beginning preparation for maturational/developmental event	**Completion** of maturational/developmental event

ing for problems and often overlook strengths. To help the reader learn to write wellness nursing diagnoses, the following section discusses common difficulties and proposed solutions. Table 2.3 summarizes this discussion.

Identification of Strengths

The belief that nurses have a place in health supervision, promote and maintain wellness activities, identify and support client strengths, and use these strengths as a foundation in times of stress is the underlying basis for wellness nursing diagnoses. Without this belief, nurses will not succeed in writing wellness diagnoses. The nurse must see the value of wellness diagnoses and be willing to make the effort to try this type of diagnosis in practice.

Table 2.3. Proposed Solutions to Difficulties in Writing Wellness Diagnoses

Difficulty	Proposed Solution
Inability to identify healthy responses	Health orientation instead of problem orientation/change in nurse values
Inability to identify contributing conditions	Comprehensive client and environmental assessment
Confusion between healthy response and goal	Process approach to wellness nursing diagnosis
Circular nursing diagnosis (similar response and condition)	Knowledge of health-related processes

Even though it may be difficult initially to identify client strengths and develop wellness diagnoses when one has been educated to identify problems and use problem-oriented diagnoses, the shift can be made. In fact, it can be fun because looking for strengths is much more optimistic than focusing on problems.

The decision about whether to use a wellness diagnosis or a problem-oriented one may be similar to looking at a glass and determining if it is half empty or half full. If the nurse expects a healthy client (a full glass) and the client has some type of illness, the nurse probably perceives the glass as half empty. However, in instances where the client is healthy but has not completely achieved a developmental task, the nurse can either perceive the glass as half empty or half full. Those nurses who lean toward terms such as *problems* or *potential problems* will see a half-empty glass. Those who identify client *strengths* and focus on *wellness* will see a glass that is half full.

Opportunities for wellness diagnoses abound in every nursing clinical specialty. Many of the activities of maternity and community health nurses involve patient teaching and health supervision for healthy, at-risk, and high-risk clients. Likewise, pediatric nurses work with children in accomplishment of age-appropriate developmental tasks regardless of whether the child is sick or well. Psychiatric nurses focus on normal developmental tasks in community health settings or when working with clients outside acute care institutions. Adult health nurses also work with clients to help them master new roles or adapt to chronic illness.

The discussion of healthy processes presented earlier will guide the nurse in looking for strengths. In addition, the wellness nursing diagnoses presented in this book and the areas for strength assessment in Chapter 3 will help the novice identify strengths and use wellness nursing diagnoses in practice. Subsequent chapters suggest healthy processes and wellness diagnoses for particular populations.

Selection of Contributing Conditions

Determining what conditions contribute to a healthy response may be difficult. Since humans are complex beings, a one-to-one relationship between a response and a condition may be very artificial. It is likely that several conditions contribute to a particular response. A clinical judgment is made to determine which condition to include in the wellness diagnosis statement.

Complete assessment of the client and environment will help identify these conditions. Client knowledge, needs, motivations, or beliefs that sustain or reinforce the healthy response are possible sources of contributing conditions.

In those instances where the healthy response is new, one or more conditions that affect the response can often be identified. However, if the strength is longstanding, such identification may be very complicated. Even though it is difficult, recognizing contributing conditions expedites goal development and provides a focus for nursing action.

When identifying conditions, the nurse must remember that the condition needs to be one where the nurse can intervene. If the condition cannot be facilitated, supported, or enhanced, there is little that the nurse can do, particularly in healthy situations. For instance, a diagnosis of *normal grief response related to death of spouse* is not useful, since the nurse can do nothing about the fact that the spouse died. However, a diagnosis of *progressive resolution of grief related to reminiscing about loved one* would be relevant because the nurse could encourage such reminiscence by asking the client to talk about or show pictures of the spouse.

Avoiding Circular Wellness Diagnoses

When two-part diagnoses are used, care must be taken to ensure that the nursing diagnosis is not circular. In a circular diagnosis, the response and the condition portions of the diagnosis are synonymous or are a part of each other. If the diagnosis is circular, goals become unclear and it is not possible to differentiate between long- and short-term goals.

To avoid a circular diagnosis, the nurse needs to be sure that the condition is not one of the cluster of health behaviors upon which the response portion of the diagnosis is based. In instances where the client must accomplish several steps before the process described in the response portion of the diagnosis is completed, the steps in the process cannot be used as the condition for the diagnosis.

Beginning maternal attachment related to establishing eye contact with the infant is an example of a circular diagnosis. Eye contact with the infant is an identifying characteristic of maternal attachment. A nursing diagnosis of *beginning maternal attachment related to increasing confidence in infant care-taking abilities* would be more useful because nursing interventions would be directed toward development of client care-taking abilities, which in turn would increase maternal attachment because of the positive feedback the mother receives from her infant during the care-taking encounters.

Likewise, *actively seeking knowledge about medical treatment or disease process related to asking questions about medications* is a circular diagnosis. The diagnosis *actively seeking knowledge*

*about medical treatment or disease process related to need to main-
tain control of health* would eliminate this problem and would
provide a basis for distinct long- and short-term goals.

In order to avoid circular diagnoses, the nurse must have
knowledge of the process the client is undergoing. Being able
to define steps of the process will help prevent inclusion of
these steps on both sides of the diagnosis.

Differentiating Responses from Goals

A major problem in writing wellness nursing diagnoses is dif-
ferentiating responses from goals. A solution for this problem,
writing responses in a process format, has been proposed. In
the past, some authors substituted positive qualifiers for negative qualifiers in the NANDA-approved diagnoses, but this
technique exacerbated the confusion between diagnosis and
goal. When words like *adequate* or *effective* replace *inadequate*
or *ineffective*, the diagnosis can be mistaken for a goal statement. In addition, if the client response is adequate or effective, is there really a need for a nursing diagnosis or nursing
care?

CASE STUDY

To illustrate the use of wellness nursing diagnosis, the
following case study is presented.

At Mary Smith's 6-week postpartum visit, the nurse
noticed the following behaviors: Mary handled her
infant with confidence when feeding and comforting
the infant, she stated that she never imagined how
much one could love a baby, and she noted that the
infant looked just like the baby's father. The nurse
remembered that Koniak-Griffin (1993) described three
components of maternal role attainment: attachment
to the infant, skill in infant care-taking and expressed
pleasure in the role. Integrating her knowledge about
maternal role with the behaviors she observed, the
nurse developed a nursing diagnosis of *beginning
attainment of maternal role.*

Although complete attainment of maternal role

was not seen, the nurse knew that the behaviors she saw were normal and appropriate for 6 weeks' postpartum. Therefore, if a problem-oriented diagnosis such as *potential problems with maternal role attainment* had been developed, the data would have been skewed, since no potential for problems was identified and all observed behaviors were within normal limits. In addition, sharing such a diagnosis with Mary could cause her to become concerned that something was wrong and a change in maternal–infant interaction might occur, resulting in the emergence of problems.

In order to develop goals for nursing care from the wellness diagnosis, the nurse determined that Mary's beginning maternal role attainment (response) was related to interacting with a healthy infant, receiving help in infant care from her husband and family, and having previous experience in infant care (conditions). The nurse and Mary discussed possible mothering role goals. Mary stated that she needed more information about infant growth and development, ways to handle future discipline matters, and new ways to incorporate her husband into the infant's care.

As a result of this discussion, a mutually satisfying long-term goal was written: Attainment of maternal role will be achieved in 9 months as evidenced by the following:

- Mary will be able to describe her infant's patterns of behavior and respond to these changing patterns in ways that will meet the baby's needs.
- Mary will continue to identify infant characteristics that remind her of family members.
- Mary and her husband will discuss ways to handle difficult care issues, such as discipline.

In order to facilitate Mary's efforts for maternal role attainment (the long-term goal), interventions were directed toward reinforcing Mary's positive caretaking behaviors, helping Mary anticipate changes in infant care that will occur as the baby grows, praising Mary and her family for the way they work together to provide infant care, and discussing ways that Mary can find time to meet her own needs as well as those of her infant. In this way, the nurse reinforced client behaviors, prepared her for the future, and facilitated conditions that fostered the development of the maternal role. As these role behaviors were reinforced, role development became stronger and the client was able to reach the long-term goal of attainment of maternal role.

SUMMARY

The focus of this chapter has been how to write a wellness nursing diagnosis. The relationship among health-related processes, nursing diagnosis, and goals has been discussed. Common problems encountered when writing wellness diagnoses, with proposed solutions, were explored. The use of a process format for the client response was emphasized in order to differentiate the diagnosis from a goal.

An attitudinal change is needed to shift from the use of problem-oriented nursing diagnoses in every situation to selecting wellness nursing diagnoses when appropriate. Although one may have difficulty in writing wellness nursing diagnoses initially, proficiency will evolve with time and experience. As the client acquires skills, achieves developmental tasks, and attains new roles, empowerment occurs. Such empowerment enhances both the client's life and the nurse's job satisfaction.

References

Koniak-Griffin, D. (1993). Maternal role attainment. *Image, 25*(3), 257–262.

Mundinger, M.O., and Jauron, G.D. (1975). Developing a nursing diagnosis. *Nursing Outlook, 23*(2), 94–98.

3
~

Assessment of Client Strengths

I n order to write wellness nursing diagnoses, client strengths must be assessed. Although nurses are quite skilled at recognizing abnormal behaviors or identifying problems, they are less adept at noting client strengths or incorporating them into client care. Since the goal of nursing education is to prepare a nurse who can problem solve and think critically, most educational experiences are directed toward development of these abilities. Consequently, clinical experiences in acute care settings are directed toward problem solving.

To facilitate nurse recognition of client strengths, a change in philosophy is needed that acknowledges the worth of noting client strengths for development of wellness nursing diagnoses. Without this change, the nurse may believe that such assessment is a waste of time and energy. The current emphasis on problem identification and cost containment in health care agencies eliminates anything that is extraneous to the central problem-oriented goal. Time is limited and is spent recording abnormal behaviors to verify the problem-oriented nursing diagnosis. Therefore, rewards must be implemented for the nurse who documents client strengths.

A variety of variables such as cultural beliefs, developmental level, cognitive ability, and moral values interact to determine whether or not a client develops particular strengths. The nurse must be aware of these influences when assessing for strengths or the nurse's own values may be super-imposed on the client.

For example, cultural values have a major influence on role assumption or role mastery attainment. Just as dominant male roles are the norm in some cultures, assertive feminine roles are not acceptable. Therefore, women from those cultures cannot be expected to be assertive, nor, in most instances, will they want to develop these traits. The nurse must not then conclude that these women have a deficit based on the nurse's beliefs in female assertiveness. Interventions to facilitate development of assertiveness would be inconsistent with client goals and cultural background.

Assessment of strengths is a relatively new field and limited literature is available on the topic. No recent literature has addressed a framework for strength assessment. Richardson and Berry (1987) suggest a strength intervention model that includes four stages: assessing, nurturing, freeing, and optimizing. Although relatively old, this model is useful when dealing with lifestyle modifications in wellness and prevention programs. It also suggests a variety of dimensions the nurse can assess to gain information about client strengths and provides motivation for nursing intervention, i.e., nurturing client strengths to facilitate adaptation to life changes.

Richardson and Berry assert that assessment of personal strengths is the first step in identifying positive health behaviors. In the second stage both the client and health care provider nurture these strengths to provide support to areas that need modification. The third stage, freeing, encourages the client to identify the healthy end of continua related to physical, social, spiritual, emotional, intellectual, and occupational dimensions. Clients then aim toward freedom from the burdens of unhealthy behaviors. The last stage, optimizing, is enhanced by development of healthy behaviors that promote the positive end of the continua described above.

On these continua, healthy behaviors are aimed at achieving "freedom from illness," "freedom from loneliness," "freedom from guilt," "freedom from hunger for love or improper display of anger or other emotions," "freedom from intellectual stagnation," and "freedom from frustration," respectively (p. 43). These six dimensions of living (physical, social, spiritual, emotional, intellectual, and occupational) could be used as a broad framework for strength assessment.

A less formal framework for general strength assessment is included in this chapter. Healthy processes for specific client populations are described in subsequent chapters. Delineation of a physical assessment is beyond the scope of this book; however, strengths in the physical/physiological area can be detected through a general physical examination. Recognition of normal physical and physiological parameters is the first step in assessing client strengths. If the client is in good overall physical health, this strength will help in coping with specific areas of dysfunction and will provide energy to accomplish maturational/developmental tasks.

~ *Areas of Strength Assessment*

The literature on wellness and health promotion focuses primarily on four areas of health promotion behavior: nutrition, physical exercise, stress reduction, and social support. Most authors assert that the outcomes of health promotion fulfill the goals of self-actualization and increased well-being. Descriptions of healthy behaviors or strengths vary from specific numbers of times exercise is practiced to types of food eaten. However, these four areas do not encompass all possible areas of strength assessment. The following paragraphs suggest a framework for strength assessment. Display 3.1 also provides a general strength assessment format. These areas are not necessarily mutually exclusive or jointly exhaustive, but are presented for consideration. The reader may collect additional data based on clinical experience.

DISPLAY 3.1.

General Strength Assessment Format

FOR THE HEALTHY OR ILL CLIENT

1. What kinds of abilities do you have to take care of your health?
2.. What kinds of things do you do to maintain or improve your health?
3. Have you made any changes in your lifestyle to improve your health in the past 2 years?
4. What goals do you have for improving your health?
5. How do you plan to go about reaching these goals?
6. What kinds of plans have you made to help you make these changes?
7. What kind of changes in your life do you see in the future?
8. Who will help you cope with these changes?
9. In the past, what did you do when you had to cope with a crisis?
10. What gives you direction in your life?

ADDITIONAL QUESTIONS
FOR THE CLIENT WHO IS ILL

11. What do you know about your illness?
12. What questions do you have about your illness?
13. What kinds of changes do you think you will have to make because of your illness?
14. How have you been able to make the changes in diet, exercise, medication, etc., that you need to make?
15. Are you comfortable with the new equipment/technology you have had to learn to use in order to take care of yourself? (If applicable)

Motivation

Participation in health care, whether it be for the purpose of promoting health, preventing disease, or coping with acute or chronic illness, begins with the client's motivation or desire to play an active role. The following questions help assess motivation:

- How does the client feel about participating in his or her care?
- Does the client wait to be told what to do by the health care provider or does the client have a plan in mind?
- Is the client capable of carrying out the plan independently?
- What are the client's short- or long-term health care goals?
- Does the client want an active part in this knowledge acquisition or does he or she prefer to be a passive recipient of health care?

Wellness or Health Promotion Behaviors

Assessing a client's general lifestyle will give patterns of healthy behaviors that are client strengths. The following questions might be useful:

- Does the client have an established program of health maintenance that includes good nutrition, physical exercise, and stress management?
- Does a consistent pattern of behaviors directed toward a healthy lifestyle emerge during assessment?
- How has the client attempted to increase healthy behaviors and decrease negative behaviors?

Nutrition

To obtain information about client nutrition, a diet history is often used. Specific data about diet habits (what is eaten, how often it is eaten, and how much is eaten) and assessment of nutritional knowledge are needed. Identifying who does the cooking in the household is useful because the client's knowledge level may be different from whoever is cooking. In the case of a male client, a wife who is motivated to change family dietary habits is a family strength. Although motivation is difficult to assess, efforts to improve dietary intake or changes taken to provide for more nutritional and balanced meals are areas of strength.

Weight maintenance or weight reduction behaviors are also part of the nutritional assessment area. In some instances, such as the anorexic client, behaviors aimed at weight gain are important for an improved health status. Helpful questions to assess nutrition include:

- Does the client know what constitutes a healthy diet?
- Can the number and type of food groupings needed per day be described?
- Does the client know how to read labels to ensure that the food purchased meets nutritional requirements?
- How closely does the client's diet follow recommended nutritional guidelines?
- What kind of dietary changes has the client made to meet recommended guidelines?
- Who cooks for the client?
- If someone other than the client does the cooking, what kind of knowledge does that person have about nutrition? About the client's specific nutritional needs?
- If the client has a prescribed diet, how closely is it followed?
- Is there a balance between intake and exercise?

In those instances where the client possesses knowledge about good nutritional habits and attempts to change nutritional practices, an appropriate wellness nursing diagnosis is

~ *Increasing knowledge about adequate nutrition*

Clients who are striving to make changes in their nutritional intake or who are eating more nutritional meals than in the past could have the wellness diagnosis

~ *Improving nutritional intake*

An appropriate diagnosis in situations where the client is consistently adhering to diet instructions would be

~ *Compliance with prescribed diet*

Stress Management

Much of the same type of information collected in the nutritional area applies to stress management. Knowledge and/or practice of stress reduction techniques, as well as awareness of sources of stress, are items the nurse might assess. Some assessment questions include:

- Does the client recognize when he or she is stressed?
- Is the client interested in information about stress reduction?
- Does the client practice any type of stress reduction techniques?
- How often are these techniques used?
- Are these techniques used correctly?

Client recognition of the factors that cause stress and modification of behavior to avoid stressful situations are strengths. Using stress reduction techniques during times of stress is also a strength. Some wellness diagnoses for this area include

~ *Increasing ability to avoid stressful situations*
~ *Beginning practice of stress management techniques*
~ *Increasing ability to maintain stress reduction through consistent use of stress management techniques*

Physical Exercise

Increasing emphasis is being given to the need for physical exercise to maintain cardiovascular wellness and prevent weight gain. The following questions are helpful:

- Does the client recognize the value of physical exercise and participate in some type of program appropriate to overall general well-being?
- Can the client determine the suitable limits (maintenance of target pulse) in order not to exceed the maximum pulse rate for age and health status?
- How frequently does the client exercise?

As clients become aware of the need for physical exercise and incorporate it into their lifestyle, these wellness diagnoses can be used:

~ *Developing goals for physical exercise*
~ *Beginning maintenance of exercise regimen*

Health-Seeking Behaviors

At the more abstract level, all the areas described in this chapter deal with the client's health-seeking behaviors. Tripp and Stachowiak (1992) describe health-seeking behaviors as those that move the client from the status quo to a positive state of health. Actively seeking information about health from experts in the health care delivery system or reading books and articles directed toward health maintenance are behaviors that help the client move toward a more positive health state. Questions that help assess strengths in this area include:

- What is the client's present level of knowledge about health promotion, or in the case of illness, knowledge about the illness?
- Does the client value being healthy?
- Does the client believe he or she is healthy?
- How eager is the client in seeking resources to gain the knowledge needed to either participate in or manage his or her care?
- Does the client have the cognitive ability to independently acquire knowledge?
- Is there motivation to improve health status?
- Is the client willing to accept responsibility for his or her own health?
- Has the client developed specific health care goals?

Clients who recognize the importance of being healthy, take responsibility for their own health status, and are motivated to gain higher levels of wellness are exhibiting strengths. Examples of wellness nursing diagnoses related to self-care or health-seeking activities are

~ *Beginning acceptance of responsibility for self-care*
~ *Accepting responsibility for self-care*
~ *Progressive identification and elimination of negative health care practices*
~ *Initiating a program of stress reduction*
~ *Actively seeking knowledge about medical treatment or disease process*

Maturational and/or Developmental Events

Clients often deal with maturational transitions (developmental tasks), role change, or situational events. Developmental crises occur at all stages of life from achieving autonomy in childhood to planning for retirement during middle age. Anticipatory planning for either maturational or transitional events reflects a client strength because it helps eliminate stress when the changes occur. Types of assessment questions for this area include:

- What maturational or transitional events does the client anticipate in the near future?
- What knowledge does the client have about the event?
- Does the client want any information about the event?
- Can the client describe how this event will change his or her lifestyle?
- What plans has the client made related to the event?

In these instances where clients have started planning for transitional events, the following examples of wellness diagnoses are useful:

~ *Beginning preparation for maturational/developmental event (specify)*
~ *Anticipating lifestyle changes required for maturational/developmental event*
~ *Learning new skills required for adaptation to developmental/maturational event*

Role Mastery

Role performance is another area where strengths can be identified. People are social beings who learn new roles and develop personal identity through feedback from others. Roles arise from relationships with people such as parents, spouses, friends, or children. Occupational roles also exist such as farmer, shop foreman, educator, policeman, or chief executive.

Illness can disturb role performance or necessitate learning new roles. However, if the client has achieved role mastery in the past, it may be possible to draw upon those strengths when learning a new role. The following questions are helpful to assess role mastery:

- What roles does the client have?
- How does the client feel when performing these roles?
- What self-expectations does the client have in these roles?
- How does the client think others perceive him or her in theses roles?

For the client who needs to learn a new role, these questions help assess plans related to the new role:

- Does the client recognize the need to plan ways to learn the new role?
- What kinds of contact has the client had with people in that role in order to observe their behaviors and/or consider whether or not those behaviors should be adopted?
- Has the client identified places where role behaviors can be safely practiced before final assumption of the role? If so, have those behaviors been practiced by the client?

A client who has learned to function well in a particular role, who finds ways to learn new roles or who continues to adjust behavior as needed to maintain role function, has strengths in the role mastery area. Wellness nursing diagnoses related to role function could center on beginning role attainment, steps in role development, or role mastery. Examples of these diagnoses include

  ~ *Planning for new role*
  ~ *Pride in ability to master new role*
  ~ *Progressive attainment of role behaviors*

Social Support

The necessity of social support has been recognized in many areas of life ranging from childbearing to cardiac rehabilitation. Clients receive emotional support from others that helps them overcome obstacles or learn new skills or behaviors. Therefore, the kind and type of social support a client has is an important component of client assessment. The following questions will help assess this area:

- Does the client live alone or with others?
- What kind of social support does the client have?
- What family members are available who can help the client deal with maturational/developmental transitions or illness?
- What kind of relationships does the client have with spouse or partner, children, and other family members?
- What other types of social networks exist (e.g., affiliation with a church, fraternal or professional organization, hobby interest club, or support group)?
- What type of affiliation does the client have with co-workers?
- Has the client developed relationships with others who are skilled in the new role he or she wants to learn?
- What sources does the client use to find answers to health-related questions?
- Does the client participate in any support groups that facilitate coping with illness or with the normal maturational crises of living?

Clients who have social support have a strength that will enable them to cope with illness or lifestyle changes. Examples of wellness nursing diagnoses related to social support include

~ *Progressive interaction with support group members*
~ *Recognizing interdependence among family members*
~ *Seeking interaction with others to learn new skill/role*

Spirituality

Spiritual strengths often help a client through the difficult times of illness or change. Assessment of these strengths goes far beyond identifying religious affiliation. Experts describe characteristics of spirituality as manifestations of joy or peace; belief in the meaning and purpose of life; and harmonious relationships with self, others, and a higher power. This spirituality often is a source of energy that enables one to cope with the conflicts and successes of daily living. The following are examples of questions a nurse might consider when assessing spirituality:

- What does the client see as his or her purpose in life?
- What beliefs, culture, or value system guide the client's actions?
- From where does the client draw emotional strength or energy to cope with life?
- Does the client have a relationship with God or believe in a higher being?
- Does the client pray or participate in any type of meditation?
- Is the client capable of self-forgiveness as well as forgiveness of others?
- What is the driving force behind the client's activities?
- What are the client's sources of satisfaction?

Most of these questions can only be answered by self-report, but the nurse can also be alert for any external signs of religious faith such as rosaries, Bibles, and prayer books. Asking the client to describe sources of strength may be one way of determining the firmness of spiritual identity or the source of energy. Knowledge of the client's philosophy of life will empower the nurse to use interventions consistent with this philosophy and/or value system.

Those clients who have a spiritual base for action regardless of particular religious beliefs, who believe in a meaning for their life, and who exhibit inner peace have spiritual strengths. Wellness nursing diagnoses related to spirituality include the following:

- ~ *Progressive religious faith*
- ~ *Maintaining strong spiritual foundation*
- ~ *Maintaining hope and trust in higher power*
- ~ *Progressive ability to forgive self and/or others*

~ *Continued belief in meaning and purpose of life*
~ *At peace with self and/or health status*

Psychological State

Assessment of feelings may also reveal particular client strengths. Feelings of self-efficacy, self-confidence, or self-esteem may restore a client's sense of adequacy in illness situations that expose vulnerability. A desire to regain or maintain control over one's health status may provide positive motivation to comply with medical treatment or learn to cope with a new lifestyle. If feelings of well-being and/or self-actualization are goals of health maintenance, health promotion, or wellness programs, these feelings need to be assessed. Some questions to consider include:

- What does the client identify as strengths and weaknesses?
- Does the client believe his or her goals have been accomplished?
- How confident is the client about the ability to do those things he or she wishes to do?
- Does the client believe in his or her own capability?
- How does the client feel about himself or herself in general?

Recognition of strengths and limitations, self-confidence, and feelings of accomplishment all reflect client strengths. Suggested wellness nursing diagnoses are

~ *Increasing desire to improve health status*
~ *Increasing ability to evaluate strengths and weaknesses in order to set realistic self-care goals*
~ *Feelings of satisfaction with past achievements*
~ *Increasing self-confidence*

Interaction with Health Care Environment

Another area for assessment is the adaptation a client makes to the health care environment. In acute care settings, clients often have to learn to live with a variety of machines such as monitors, pumps that regulate intravenous fluids, and ventilators. Due to short hospital stays, clients may go home with central lines for parenteral nutrition, chemotherapy, or other types of medication. Infants may be connected to apnea monitors and women at risk for premature labor may use fetal monitors at home for detecting the presence of contractions.

Any of these situations demands orientation to the equipment, knowledge of resources about who to call in the event of monitor failure or equipment malfunction, and changes in lifestyle to accommodate the presence of such equipment. Although some of the equipment is indicated for specific diseases, other equipment may simply monitor a high-risk situation. In any instance, the client may have strengths that allow smooth adaptation to these intrusions in routine activities of daily living. Assessment questions include:

- Does the client understand the purpose for the equipment?
- Does the client know how to use the equipment?
- Does the client know where to get help if needed?
- Is the client comfortable with the equipment?
- What kinds of changes has the client made in order to incorporate the equipment into his or her lifestyle?

Ability to describe how equipment is used, relative ease in handling the equipment, and knowledge of where to obtain help if needed are client strengths in this area. Examples of wellness nursing diagnoses include

~ *Beginning skill in use of medical equipment/technology (specify)*

~ *Modifying home environment to accommodate medical technology*

Compliance

In working with clients who are receiving medical care, the nurse assesses how well they are able to follow the instructions given with prescribed medications, diet, or other types of treatments. To assess knowledge and motivation, the nurse reviews with the client any information received from the physician or other health care providers. Some questions that could be asked include:

- Does the client know why particular drugs have been pre-scribed, when these drugs should be taken, and the side effects?
- Can the client understand the limitations or restrictions of a particular diet?
- Is the client willing to accept those restrictions?
- What specifics about the client's lifestyle facilitate ability to follow prescribed medication, diet, etc.?

Resources may include not only money for drugs and supplies, but also access to transportation or physical assistance with tasks of daily living. In those instances where the client is fol-lowing the instructions that have been given, wellness nurs-ing diagnoses might be

~ *Increasing compliance with prescribed treatment*
~ *Motivation to follow prescribed medical treatment*

Coping Skills

Another area of client strengths is the coping skills used to deal with stress, illness, or the hassles of everyday living. Some of these skills may overlap with those mentioned in the stress reduction and spiritual areas. Techniques of stress management, meditation, and prayer are examples of coping skills. In addi-tion, scheduled time for relaxation or privacy, feelings of hope, or actions to alter the source of stress are all ways of coping.

Some clients will endeavor to obtain as much information about an event as possible in order to cope with the accom-panying stress; others prefer not to have any information. Assessment questions for this area include:

- How does the client usually deal with problems?
- What successes has the client had in the past?
- Does the client believe the strategies he or she usually uses will work in this situation?

- Does the client have a variety of coping strategies to allow flexibility under stress?

Having a variety of coping strategies to use in stressful situations is a client strength. Use of coping skills and past ability to cope with stress also are client strengths. Examples of wellness nursing diagnoses would be

~ *Ongoing use of coping skills*
~ *Demonstrated ability to cope with stress*

Personal Success/Mastery

No assessment of strengths seems complete without identifying those areas where the client feels success has been achieved. In this instance, the client's perception is what determines the amount or type of success. What type of things does the client feel have been mastered? Areas of mastery pertain to learning a skill such as diagnosis and repair of motor vehicles, completing a task such as writing a report or making a piece of furniture, or being recognized as an expert in a particular field of work.

Recognizing past successes provides hope for success in the future. In the case of illness, past success may help the client recognize that personal strengths are available to cope with the present illness. A nursing diagnosis in this area is probably not necessary, but discussion of those successes will foster self-esteem and hope, or lessen feelings of vulnerability.

The preceding paragraphs involve a general assessment of strengths. Display 3.1 includes some questions the nurse can ask the client to begin a strength assessment. Using interviewing skills, the nurse can elicit a great deal of information with these questions.

Since a mere listing of representative diagnoses for each area may not be helpful, Table 3.1 (see overleaf) includes some behaviors indicative of most of the diagnoses listed above as well as some interventions to nurture these strengths.

SUMMARY

To help the nurse assess client strengths, a variety of areas that will provide an overall general assessment have been discussed in this chapter. Examples of wellness nursing diagnoses relevant to these areas have also been given. As a complement to this general assessment, subsequent chapters will discuss health-related processes for particular populations that provide further information for strength assessment and development of wellness diagnoses.

References

Richardson, G.E., and Berry, N.F. (1987). Strength intervention: An approach to lifestyle modification. *Health Education*, *18*(3), 42–206.

Tripp, S.L., and Stachowiak, B. (1992). Health maintenance, health promotion: Is there a difference? *Public Health Nursing*, 9, 155–161.

Table 3.1. Relationships Among Selected Wellness Nursing Diagnoses, Behaviors, and Interventions

Area	Wellness Nursing Diagnosis	Client Behaviors	Nursing Interventions
Nutrition	*Increasing knowledge about adequate nutrition*	Describes daily intake that satisfies ADA minimum daily requirements	Reinforce knowledge
			Give positive reinforcement for good nutritional behaviors
		Uses diet recall to report a diet that is nutritionally sound	Clarify misunderstandings
	Improving nutritional intake	Reviews diet history to reveal better balance between food groups and increase or decrease in caloric intake as appropriate	Give positive reinforcement for improvement
			Explore ways diet can be improved
			Provide food options that would increase nutritional intake (less fat, more fiber, balance of food groups, etc.)
	Compliance with prescribed diet	Describes diet restrictions	Reinforce compliance
		Follows diet as directed	Clarify any misunderstandings

Stress management	*Increasing ability to avoid stressful situations*	Describes sources of stress and can state ways to avoid these situations	Reinforce stress management behaviors
			Discuss ways to reduce stress if it cannot be avoided
		Recognizes own physical and psychological response to stress	
	Beginning practice of stress management techniques	Reports types of stress management techniques used and states they are used intermittently	Reinforce relaxation behaviors
			Provide alternative methods of stress management
		Demonstrates ability to relax while using relaxation techniques	Explore factors that impede or facilitate use of relaxation
	Increasing ability to maintain stress reduction through consistent use of stress management techniques	Same as above but has frequent use (3–5 times/week)	Praise use of stress management techniques
			Explore factors that impede or facilitate use of relaxation
Exercise	*Developing goals for physical exercise*	Reports interest and motivation to start an exercise program	Reinforce interest in exercise
			Suggest ways to obtain exercise

(continued)

51

Area	Wellness Nursing Diagnosis	Client Behaviors	Nursing Interventions
Exercise (cont'd.)	*Developing goals for physical exercise (cont'd.)*	Outlines plan to start exercise program	Help develop plan to begin exercise program
		Describes chosen exercise regimen	Discuss ways to increase exercise
	Beginning maintenance of exercise regimen	Reports use of exercise regimen 1–2 times/week	Explore factors that facilitate or impede exercise
Health-seeking behaviors	*Beginning acceptance of responsibility for self-care*	Discusses interest in increasing own responsibility for self-care	Reinforce interest in self-care
			Suggest courses of action directed at developing healthy lifestyle
	Accepting responsibility for self-care	Describes ways to carry out independent health care practices to promote healthy lifestyle (such as nutrition, exercise, stress management, etc.)	Reinforce healthy lifestyle behaviors
	Progressive identification and elimination of negative health care practices	Describes negative health care practices	Praise efforts for self-care
		Sets goal to eliminate at least one negative health care practice	Explore factors that help or hinder goal achievement

52

Initiating a program of stress reduction	Recognizes what things cause stress	Help client identify signs and symptoms of stress
	Recognizes when stressed	Explain methods of stress reduction and discuss pros and cons of each method
	Discusses methods of stress reduction	Assist client in selecting methods that fit into lifestyle
	Selects methods that can be used	
	Discusses how stress reduction techniques can be integrated into life	
Actively seeking knowledge about medical treatment or disease process	Asks questions about treatment or disease process	Reinforce knowledge
	Seeks and reads written material about treatment or disease process	Reinforce ability to ask health care professionals questions about treatment or disease process
	Describes relationships between disease process and treatment as appropriate	Provide information about treatment or disease process in oral, written, or audiovisual format

(continued)

Area	Wellness Nursing Diagnosis	Client Behaviors	Nursing Interventions
Health-seeking behaviors (cont'd.)	*Actively seeking knowledge about medical treatment or disease process (cont'd.)*	Discusses activities specific to disease that will improve health status	Discuss ways that client can improve health
Maturational/ developmental events	*Beginning preparation for maturational/developmental event (specify)*	Seeks knowledge through attendance at classes and/or reading widely about event	Provide resources that explain transitional changes
			Help prioritize use of resources
			Reinforce decision to prepare for event
	Anticipating lifestyle changes required for maturational/developmental event	Describes expectations of the event	Reinforce correct information
		Describes feelings related to the anticipated changes	Correct misinformation
			Use role-play or other techniques to provide practice in lifestyle changes
	Learning new skills required for adaptation to developmental/ maturational event	Explains or demonstrates the new skills learned	Provide resources that describe needed skills
		Identifies social support for learn-	Explore ways to learn new skills

		ing new skill	Request demonstration of new skills as appropriate
Role mastery	Planning for new role	Attends classes, reads about role, discusses ways new role will affect lifestyle	Help identify new behavior/skills needed
			Provide resources where client can gain new information or skills related to new role
			Reinforce learning activities
	Pride in ability to master new role	Identifies role mastery behaviors	Help client identify accomplishments and role behaviors
		Describes accomplishments resulting from new role	Praise accomplishments
	Progressive attainment of role behaviors	Describes beginning feelings of confidence and accomplishment related to role	Explore ways to identify role attainment
		Identifies and/or demonstrates new role behaviors	Reinforce behaviors

(continued)

Area	Wellness Nursing Diagnosis	Client Behaviors	Nursing Interventions
Role mastery (cont'd.)	*Progressive attainment of role behaviors (cont'd.)*		Use role-play and other techniques to help client gain new behaviors
			Discuss factors that facilitate or impede role attainment
Social support	*Progressive interaction with support group members*	Reports attendance at support group	Provide resources about specific support groups
		Describes experiences in support group	Explore and reinforce ways support groups have helped client cope
			Reinforce support group interaction
	Recognizing interdependence among family members	Describes help received from family members to reach goal	Explore ways family members have facilitated goal attainment
		Reviews how goal was reached	Reinforce family interaction
	Seeking interaction with others to learn new skill/role	Describes observing others who have the type of skill/role needed	Suggest possible sources for learning skill/role from peers

		in order to gain knowledge	Reinforce social interaction
		Discusses or demonstrates learned skill/role	Reinforce or correct skill/role behaviors as appropriate
		States that peer learning is beneficial and is grateful to others for sharing their skill/role behaviors	
Spiritual	*Progressive religious faith*	Describes value/belief system	Reinforce religious practices
		Describes role faith has in helping cope with life/illness	Referrals to clergy as appropriate
	Maintaining strong spiritual foundation	Demonstrates consistent pattern of church attendance, prayer, and/or Bible study	Reinforce behaviors
		Describes value/belief system	If needed, give information about religious services, clergy, etc.
	Maintaining hope and trust in higher power	Describes ways hope has helped in the past	Encourage description of past experiences where hope has helped in coping
		Describes realistic hope in spite of illness	

(continued)

57

Area	Wellness Nursing Diagnosis	Client Behaviors	Nursing Interventions
Spiritual (cont'd.)	Maintaining hope and trust in higher power (cont'd.)	Describes source of hope or trust	Reinforce realistic hope Encourage reliance on personal beliefs
	Progressive ability to forgive self and/or others	Acknowledges that everyone makes mistakes	Reinforce idea that no one is perfect
		Recognizes need to forgive self and/or others	Encourage discussion of past or present events where forgiveness is desired
		Accepts forgiveness from others	Be objective, nonjudgmental
			Role model forgiveness
			Reinforce ability to forgive self and/or others
	Continued belief in meaning and purpose of life	Asserts belief that life has meaning and purpose	Encourage discussion of belief
			Reinforce beliefs
		Describes ways that life has meaning and purpose	Reinforce ways client describes that life has meaning and purpose

	At peace with self and/or health status	Expresses satisfaction with belief system	Reinforce behaviors
		Exhibits calmness in difficult situation	Provide encouragement
Psychological	*Increasing desire to improve health status*	Self-report of desire to improve health status	Explore possibilities of how to improve health status
		Identifies behaviors that can be changed to improve health status	Reinforce motivation
			Discuss factors that will help or impede goal attainment
	Increasing ability to evaluate personal strengths and weaknesses in order to set realistic self-care goals	States strengths and weaknesses	Help formulate plan for goal attainment
		Chooses one or more weaknesses to eliminate if possible	Explore ways that strengths and weaknesses will affect goal attainment
		States self-care goals	Discuss ways to overcome identified weakness

(continued)

Area	Wellness Nursing Diagnosis	Client Behaviors	Nursing Interventions
Psychological (cont'd.)	*Feelings of satisfaction with past achievements*	Describes feelings of satisfaction	Reinforce feelings of satisfaction
		Discusses past accomplishments	Relate past accomplishments to present and future situations in order to provide hope for success
	Increasing self-confidence	Describes feelings of increased self-confidence	Provide evidence of behaviors that reflect increased self-confidence
		Identifies factors that have contributed to increased self-confidence	Encourage reflection on achievements
			Reinforce feelings of self-confidence
Interaction with health care environment	*Beginning skill in use of medical equipment/technology (specify)*	States reason for medical equipment/technology	Reinforce knowledge
			Clarify misconceptions
		Describes correct use of equipment/technology	Demonstrate correct use of equipment/technology
		Lists advantages and/or disadvantages of equipment/technology	Watch client use equipment/

	Demonstrates proper use of equipment/technology	technology and reinforce accuracies while correcting mistakes
	Handles equipment with relative ease	
Modifying home environment to accommodate medical technology		
	Provides space for equipment/technology	Reinforce modifications
	Placement of equipment/technology provides easy access	Discuss alternative placement as appropriate
	Placement of equipment/technology allows for electrical safety, if appropriate, as well as physical safety	Suggest other alternatives as appropriate
Compliance	States purpose of treatment and explains treatment plan to be followed	Reinforce knowledge/compliance behaviors
Increasing compliance with prescribed treatment	Follows treatment as prescribed—amount, time, method, etc., as appropriate	Answer questions or explain why treatment is needed

(continued)

Area	Wellness Nursing Diagnosis	Client Behaviors	Nursing Interventions
Compliance (cont'd.)	*Increasing compliance with prescribed treatment (cont'd.)*	Continues to seek/gain information about treatment	Discuss expectations of treatment and reinforce those that are realistic
		Explains reasons why treatment is ordered	Support lifestyle changes that may be necessary to incorporate medical treatment into daily routine
		Adjusts lifestyle to fit treatment regimen	
		Discusses expectations of treatment	
	Motivation to follow prescribed medical treatment	States need for treatment	Reinforce knowledge
		Describes personal reasons why treatment should be followed	Praise motivation
		Identifies factors that help or hinder compliance	Discuss ways to facilitate action/compliance
Coping skills	*Ongoing use of coping skills*	Values use of coping skills when feeling stressed	Reinforce use of coping skills
			Explore alternative coping skills

Demonstrated ability to cope with stress	Describes coping skills used when in a stressful situation	Praise successful outcomes/ behavioral changes
	Provides evidence that use of coping skills changes behaviors such as (a) demonstrates relaxation, (b) can lower blood pressure through biofeedback, etc.	Praise efforts to cope
		Encourage continued use of coping skills
		Explore alternative ways to deal with stress

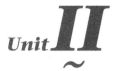

Unit *II*
~

*W*ellness Nursing Diagnosis
Across the Lifespan

~

4

~

Wellness Nursing Diagnoses for the Childbearing Family

In most instances, the childbearing cycle is a normal maturational process that occurs with a positive outcome—a healthy baby. This chapter will deal only with the normal processes of childbearing. Entire books have been written on high-risk pregnancy and examples of problem-oriented nursing diagnoses are plentiful. Conversely, little is written about wellness nursing diagnoses for the normal childbearing year.

In a normal pregnancy or a high-risk one, the goal is to provide as normal an outcome as possible. Thus, even in high-risk situations, the nurse's goal is to empower clients so that they are competent, confident parents. With clients who experience high-risk pregnancies, wellness diagnoses may be useful in those areas of the pregnancy that are within normal limits. Recognizing that they have normal aspects to their pregnancy can help these women mobilize their strengths to deal with the abnormal components.

~ *Assessment of Strengths*

In formulating wellness nursing diagnoses, specific childbearing processes must be assessed to identify client strengths. These processes are different from the areas identified in

Chapter 3 and supplement the general assessment of strengths that can be used for any adult. In this chapter, some questions are given to help the nurse assess the pregnant woman, but they are not intended to be all-inclusive.

As mentioned previously, the nurse assesses the client's response and any contributing factors (conditions) influencing that response. Many factors will influence responses to pregnancy including cultural beliefs and practices; age; educational level; socioeconomic status; past experiences with pregnancy; history of medical problems; relationships with health care providers; and fears, anxieties, and/or expectations of pregnancy and childbirth.

The examples of wellness nursing diagnoses given in this chapter deal with the first half of the diagnosis (response of the client). The second part of the diagnosis (condition) will vary depending on the contributing factors identified by the nurse and are not included in the examples.

Since the pregnant woman is the client most frequently seen during pregnancy, assessment data about the expectant father's feelings or about integration of the family are often obtained from the pregnant woman and thus are screened through her eyes. Some examples of wellness nursing diagnoses presented here will pertain to the expectant mother, some to either the pregnant woman or her partner, and others to the expectant father. However, most diagnoses will deal with the pregnant woman. Wellness nursing diagnoses for the neonate are also included.

Using Developmental Tasks of the Childbearing Year for Wellness Diagnoses

Although minor variations exist among authors, many books describe the developmental tasks of pregnancy. Colman and Colman (1991) declare that there are six developmental tasks for the childbearing year: (1) to accept the pregnancy; (2) to accept the reality of the fetus; (3) to reevaluate the older generation of parents; (4) to reevaluate the relationship between partners; (5) to accept the baby as a separate person; and (6) to integrate the parental identity (pp. 199–219). Although presented as discrete entities, in reality these tasks often overlap.

Expectant fathers attend to the developmental tasks of pregnancy at different times than expectant mothers. Since the woman experiences physical and physiological changes, she is much more attuned to the pregnancy than is the expectant father and may undertake the developmental tasks earlier in pregnancy.

In a classic article about fathering, May (1982) reports three phases of father involvement during pregnancy. The first, the announcement phase, occurs early in pregnancy and is a time of joy if the man desires the pregnancy. However, after the initial excitement about being pregnant, he remains fairly uninvolved with the pregnancy and enters the moratorium phase. This lack of interest on the part of the father may be in direct conflict with concerns of the expectant mother who needs reassurance and support from her partner as she experiences physical and emotional changes. However, the moratorium ends once the pregnancy becomes visible.

The last phase, the focusing phase, is a time when the pregnancy becomes real and important in the man's life. During this time, he starts dealing with the role changes inherent in being a father, evaluates the type of fathering he experienced, and begins prenatal paternal–infant attachment.

When considering wellness nursing diagnoses for childbearing, the developmental tasks are an appropriate place to begin. One could have a diagnosis of *accomplishing the developmental tasks of childbearing*. However, this seems very global and would communicate little to other health care providers. Therefore, each developmental task will be addressed in the following paragraphs in order to identify more specific wellness diagnoses.

Accepting the Pregnancy   Not only must the pregnancy be accepted, but the mother must deal with the changes that occur as a result of it. She will need to find medical care, she will experience physical changes that may impede her usual routine, and her role as a woman will be redefined because of her pregnancy. Without initial acceptance, the woman will be unable to proceed with the other developmental tasks unique to pregnancy.

Key questions the nurse might consider when assessing whether this developmental task has been accomplished include:

- Is the woman receiving prenatal care and when did this begin?
- What kind of statements does the woman make about her pregnancy?
- Does the woman seem excited about this pregnancy?
- What does she tell others about her pregnancy?

Behaviors that indicate acceptance of the pregnancy include seeking medical care to determine that the pregnancy does exist, recognizing that she is ambivalent about being pregnant even though she wants a baby, expressing feelings of excitement about the upcoming event, and sharing the fact that she is pregnant with others. Wellness nursing diagnoses related to this task include

- *Beginning acceptance of reality of the pregnancy*
- *Seeking early prenatal care*
- *Increasing joy about being pregnant*

The first and third diagnoses listed above could also apply to the expectant father.

As the pregnancy progresses, many physical and psychological changes take place due to hormonal influences on the body. During the second or third trimesters, some of these changes may necessitate changes in lifestyle. For instance, due to weight gain and displacement of her center of gravity, the woman may have difficulty getting up from a chair or getting out of bed. As a result, she may have to get up at the same time her husband does regardless of former sleep patterns.

Body-space relationships change and the pregnant woman must adjust to an increased girth. Thus, it may be difficult for her to reach items in out-of-the-way places, get through tight spaces, or tie her own shoes. Maternity clothes indicate to all the world that she is pregnant and strangers may pat her abdomen. Body image changes occur. Pregnant women frequently express concern that their weight gain makes them unattractive.

Assessing how the woman accepts these changes gives the nurse some idea of how well the woman is accepting the pregnancy and if she is coping with the normal changes of pregnancy. Questions that a nurse might consider include:

- What kinds of physical changes is the woman having?
- What kind of adaptation is she making to these changes?
- How does the woman feel about her changing size?

A wellness nursing diagnosis related to these normal physiological changes would be

~ *Progressive incorporation of physical changes of pregnancy into lifestyle*

Accepting the Reality of the Fetus

Even before birth, parents start to develop a relationship with the unborn child. Listening to fetal heart tones or watching an ultrasound of fetal movement helps parents to recognize the existence of the fetus. Even early in pregnancy, couples may pick out names or begin to acquire things for the baby. As the pregnancy progresses, the mother may start calling the fetus by name, may identify particular fetal characteristics such as "this is an active baby," or may point out fetal parts. Questions the nurse might consider related to this developmental task include:

- Has the woman seen an ultrasound of her fetus? How did she react when she saw it?
- Has she heard the fetal heartbeat?
- Has she begun to think about items she needs for the baby? If so, has she bought them, considered where to buy them, or made a list?
- Does she call the fetus by name or point out particular fetal parts such as feet or elbows?

Wellness diagnoses related to this developmental task include

~ *Progressive acceptance of reality of the fetus*
~ *Beginning preparation of environment (nesting) for new infant*
~ *Beginning prenatal attachment*

Any of these diagnoses could apply to the expectant father as well as the pregnant woman.

Reevaluating the Older Generation of Parents   As expectant parents start to consider their role as parents, they remember the kind of parenting they received. From their parents' role modeling, they select the parenting behaviors they wish to continue and discard behaviors they do not like. The outcome of this evaluation will be acceptance of both the adequacies and inadequacies in parenting received as a child.

Appreciation for the parents' struggles will develop and the pregnant woman will assume a more equal role with her mother as the pregnancy progresses. She will also recognize that she has to establish her own mothering role and conflicts may arise between that role and the one her mother assumes. Ultimately, those conflicts will have to be resolved before the new family can assume parenting roles independent from the older generation. Some assessment questions include:

- What kind of relationship does the client have with her mother?
- Has the woman thought about what kind of mother she would like to be?
- Which mothering behaviors does she want to adopt?
- Which mothering behaviors does she reject?

A wellness diagnosis related to this developmental task is

~ *Examining relationship with own mother*

Reevaluating the Relationship Between Partners   As additions to the couple in a first pregnancy or to the existing family are contemplated, changes in that family constellation are recognized. Both parents begin to realize that the new baby will create changes in their life. They also become aware of their interdependence and wonder if their partner will still have time for them.

If they choose to attend prepared childbirth classes, they may struggle to become a team who will work together during labor. Fantasizing about the type of parent one's partner will be also occurs. The need to develop a cohesive bond that sustains and maintains each other during the difficult times of pregnancy and parenting becomes evident. Assessment questions might include:

- Has the couple thought about the changes that will occur in their life as a result of having a baby?
- What kind of changes do they predict?
- What kind of parent do they think their spouse will make?
- How will they find time to meet their own needs and their needs as a couple?
- How well do they work together practicing breathing and relaxation exercises for labor?

As couples work through this developmental task, some wellness nursing diagnoses include

~ Developing a working relationship directed toward mutual support during pregnancy and parenting
~ Recognizing family interdependence

Obviously, these diagnoses can be considered for both partners.

Acceptance of the Infant as a Separate Person   This task begins in the latter part of pregnancy. Just as the pregnant woman recognized the fetus as a part of her body early in pregnancy, she now prepares for separation from that fetus during the upcoming labor.

It is not uncommon for the couple to fantasize about what the infant will look like as well as what type of personality the child will have. Pregnant couples often describe their fetus in terms of appearance, temperament, gender, sleep/wake cycle, and ability to communicate. In addition, couples attribute meaning to fetal behaviors. Multigravid couples compare the present fetus with fetal experiences from other pregnancies. The ability to discern fetal behavior as well as to describe its meaning, and to interact with the fetus during the third trimester, demonstrates progressive separation of the fetus from the mother.

Other evidence of acceptance of an infant as a separate person involves preparation for the infant's arrival. Designation of a room for the nursery and subsequent decorating of that room, shopping for baby clothes, and attendance at baby showers are also behaviors that indicate anticipation of the infant.

With birth, new parents have to give up the fantasy of the perfect baby they expected and accept the infant they received. Even parents who have normal infants may have fantasized about a beautiful baby who does not cry. Newborns, on the other hand, are red, wrinkled, crying beings.

Whatever prenatal attachment has occurred will blossom into a fully developed attachment with the newborn. Bonding is a process that evolves into a specific, long-lasting relationship. This process is reciprocal between the parent and infant. It occurs when each person contributes behaviors that reinforce the process and when the two persons are physically close to each other.

Assessment questions vary across the specific time of childbearing, but might include:

- What kinds of fantasies does the woman have about the fetus?
- How does she compare this fetus with experiences in previous pregnancies?
- How does she interact with the fetus?
- What clothing, equipment, or toys does she have for the baby?
- Has she planned a room for the baby?
- Has she had any baby showers, received any baby gifts, or requested any specific items for the baby?
- How is the baby similar to the one she expected?
- What attachment behaviors does she exhibit with the

baby—holding the infant *en face,* talking to the baby, calling the baby by name, identifying infant characteristics that are similar to other family members, etc.?

For this task, wellness nursing diagnoses include

~ *Beginning fantasies about the infant's personality*
~ *Beginning maternal–infant attachment*
~ *Resolving conflict between fantasized infant and actual infant*

These diagnoses can be modified for the new father.

Integration of the Parental Identity Development of maternal role begins early in pregnancy and continues for at least a year postpartum (Mercer, 1985). Rubin (1967) maintains that this process of role acquisition is continuous and has three stages: taking-in, taking-on, and letting-go. She describes the operations involved in this process as mimicry, role-play, fantasy, introjection-projection-rejection, and grief work (p. 240).

Initially, the pregnant woman mimics others she has seen in the role. For example, she dresses for the role in maternity clothes, she eats what she has read pregnant women should eat, or she follows whatever traditions her culture prescribes for pregnant women. In order to prepare herself for the role, she may seek opportunities to give child care, such as in day care centers or church nurseries.

During this time, she may fantasize about what she believes a "good" mother to be. As she becomes aware of role models in her environment, she observes their mothering behaviors and selects the ones she wishes to incorporate into her own role. Grief work refers to giving up or modifying old roles in preparation for acceptance of the new role.

To assess how well the woman is progressing in attainment of maternal role, the following questions could be asked:

- Has the woman selected particular behaviors that she thinks a pregnant woman should exhibit (e.g., eating spe-

cific foods, deleting caffeine and alcohol from her diet, incorporating culture-specific activities into her lifestyle)?
- Has the woman chosen any mothering behaviors she wants to develop? If so, what are they?
- What kinds of fantasies does she have about her ability to be a mother?
- If needed, has she found ways to increase her knowledge of newborns?
- What behaviors and/or roles does she recognize she will have to give up?

Suggested wellness nursing diagnoses related to maternal role behaviors are

~ *Beginning attainment of maternal role*
~ *Integrating fantasy role with actual mothering role*

New fathers may go through much the same process, even though they have different behaviors, when they are acquiring the paternal role.

Wellness Nursing Diagnoses for Labor

Although not specifically identified in the developmental tasks of pregnancy, the pregnant woman must also experience labor. How well she prepares for this event will ultimately influence how well she copes with the experience. Some women wish to control as many aspects of their labor as possible whereas others are content to be passive.

Attendance at prepared childbirth classes, reading books and articles about labor, and talking to others about their labor experiences are all ways one can learn about what to expect. Evaluation of how well the woman uses coping techniques such as breathing, relaxation, or use of medication during labor also provides data for wellness nursing diagnoses. Assessment questions might include:

- What kinds of things has the woman done to prepare herself for labor (e.g., attended childbirth classes, read books, asked questions of other women and/or health care professionals)?

- How well can the woman use relaxation techniques and breathing exercises?
- What are the woman's expectations about labor?
- What would the woman like to be able to do during labor?

Wellness diagnoses related to labor and preparation for labor are

~ *Progressive preparation for labor*
~ *Creating a labor plan to communicate personal desires for labor experience*
~ *Maintaining control during labor*

In terms of labor preparation, the expectant father may be an active or inactive participant depending on the wishes of the couple. A wellness diagnosis for an expectant father would be

~ *Acquiring role of labor coach*

Wellness Nursing Diagnoses for Postpartum

After the baby is born, the new mother must develop confidence in her infant care skills. The previous paragraphs about maternal role also apply postpartum. Additionally, success in infant feeding is necessary. Mothers may elect to breastfeed or bottle-feed.

One wellness nursing diagnosis related to breastfeeding in the literature is *effective breastfeeding,* which is defined as "the state in which a mother–infant dyad/family exhibits adequate proficiency and satisfaction with breastfeeding process neonate, or family exhibits proficiency and satisfaction with breast-feeding process" (NANDA, 1994, p. 67). Breastfeeding is a process that is learned over time. Since breastfeeding involves a nursing couple, both mothers and neonates must learn to breastfeed.

Assessment of breastfeeding would include observation of mother and infant. Examples of questions that could be used for assessment include:

- Is the infant swallowing milk?
- In what positions can the mother breastfeed comfortably?
- How well is the infant latched on to the breast?

- Does the mother express satisfaction with breastfeeding?
- Is the infant gaining weight?
- Is the infant well hydrated?

If the process is proceeding as expected and success is predicted even though the process is not completed, a wellness diagnosis could be

~ *Beginning establishment of breastfeeding*

Other child care skills such as handling the infant, being able to soothe the infant in distress, bathing, and diapering must be acquired. In order to feel adequate as a mother, the woman needs to feel confident in these areas. Positive feedback from the infant will enhance these feelings of confidence. Assessment could include the following questions:

- How well does the mother handle the infant?
- Does the mother know how to control the infant's head?
- How does the mother describe the meaning of the infant's cries?
- Does the mother feel comfortable when bathing her infant, when changing diapers, and when feeding her infant?
- How realistic are the mother's expectations of her infant?
- How does the infant respond to the mother's touch?

A wellness nursing diagnosis for this situation is

~ *Increasing confidence in infant care skills*

New fathers also need to develop infant care skills. However, the mother is often the gatekeeper who determines how frequently, and in what way, the father is involved in child care. Therefore, the nurse will encourage the mother to find ways to involve the father in the baby's care. The above diagnosis would also be appropriate for a new father.

Another task for the childbearing family is to integrate the infant into the family. Multiparous women often express concern about how well other children in the family will accept the new baby. Suggestions about ways to reduce the amount of sibling rivalry are frequently sought by pregnant women. Recognition that the infant is part of the family, incorporation of the infant's needs and schedules into everyday living, and acceptance of the new infant by other children are all means by which the infant is integrated into the family structure. Some questions for assessment would include:

- How do other children interact with the infant?
- Do the parents or other family members recognize family characteristics in the infant's looks or actions? If so, what are they?
- How smoothly are family activities continuing with the appearance of the new baby?
- What kinds of adaptations has the family made since the birth of the baby?

An appropriate wellness nursing diagnosis would be

~ *Beginning integration of the infant into the family*

In today's world, women often perform multiple roles such as wife, mother, and career woman. The woman who plans to return to work outside the home has to balance her need to maintain a career and the need to give full-time care to her infant. Reorganizing time allocation, setting priorities, integrating the mothering role into her identity, and finding child care facilities are just a few of the things the woman must accomplish prior to her return to work. The first few months at work may be a challenge as these multiple roles blend into a whole. Assessment questions could include:

- What are the woman's expectations of herself within her multiple roles?
- How well can the woman combine activities in order to meet her role demands?
- Can the woman "let go" of some activities in order to meet the needs of herself, her infant, and her family?
- If returning to work, what plans for child care have been made?
- How easy is it for the woman to rearrange priorities?

A wellness nursing diagnosis in this situation could be

~ *Beginning adjustment to multiple roles*

Wellness Nursing Diagnoses for the Neonate

The first step the infant must take is adjustment to extrauterine life. Many physiological changes occur during this adjustment. Additionally, the infant experiences various stages of sleep and activity ranging from regular sleep to awake and crying states that affect the baby's response to the surrounding world. Although comprehensive physical assessment of the infant is beyond the scope of this book, some normal physiological and interactive processes will be briefly discussed.

Adjustment to extrauterine life involves needs for oxygen, nutrition, temperature regulation, and safety. Additionally, new infants need the ability to comfort themselves and to elicit caretaking behaviors from parents or caregivers. Examples of physiologic wellness nursing diagnoses include

~ *Adequate oxygen exchange*
~ *Maintenance of thermoregulation*
~ *Adequate nutritional intake*

Although it has been suggested that use of the word *adequate* may contribute to a vague nursing diagnosis, this adjective seems appropriate when dealing with physiologic response.

Adequate oxygen exchange is dependent on normal lung functioning. In order to achieve an adequate nutritional intake, the infant must be able to suckle, to digest formula or breast milk, and to elicit feeding behaviors from caretakers at appropriate times. Maintenance of thermoregulation in a normal newborn depends primarily on the caretaker, who must provide a warm environment that prevents heat loss. If the infant is coping well with life outside the womb and is able to meet oxygen demands, maintain a normal body temperature, and successfully adapt to stimuli, a useful wellness diagnosis would be

~ *Progressive transition to extrauterine life*

When assessing newborns, one must not only observe the infant's behaviors, but must also assess the maternal–infant interaction. This interaction has a profound influence on the life of a newborn for it determines, in many ways, how well his or her needs are met. By maintaining or avoiding eye contact during the alert state, the infant effectively stimulates or eradicates social interaction. This interaction is influenced by the maturity of the infant and the attributes of the mother (Walker, 1992, p. 315). Infants react to their mother's voice, move in response to the rhythm of their mother's speech, and remain attuned to their mother's behavior since they have not yet recognized their existence apart from their mother. Over the first few weeks of life, the nurse can assess for this ability to regulate social interaction. Not only can these data be used to help the mother learn about her particular infant, but the nurse can also determine if the infant has these skills.

Assessment of the mother–infant interaction might include the following questions:

- Does the infant look at its mother when she talks?
- At what times does the infant turn away from the mother or caregiver?
- Does the mother hold the infant *en face*?
- Can the mother recognize when the infant has been overstimulated?
- What does the mother do if the infant has been overstimulated?
- Does the mother recognize the difference between infant cries in order to determine different needs?

If the mutual interaction between infant and mother is going smoothly—i.e., the mother is attuned to her infant's needs and the infant is able to send cues that indicate a need is present or a need has been met—a wellness diagnosis would be

~ *Progressive synchrony with mother*

The infant who can elicit caretaking behaviors will have his or her needs met better than the one who cannot elicit such behaviors. For instance, infants who smile and respond to a voice provide a reward for the person interacting with them. The mother also receives positive feedback when her infant feeds well. Depending on the age of the infant, the nurse might consider the following questions for assessment:

- Does the infant maintain eye contact?
- If able to smile, does the infant respond to the caregiver with a smile?
- How well does the infant feed? Are the infant's behaviors different with different caretakers?
- Does the infant express excitement at seeing the caregiver?

A wellness nursing diagnosis in this instance would be

~ *Beginning to elicit caretaking behaviors*

Habituation to stimuli, ability to provide self-comfort when upset, and ability to smile and cuddle are assessment components of how an infant responds to stimuli. This assessment should be done in various states of awareness to provide the mother with clues about her infant's patterns of behavior. The infant's ability to self-regulate impacts his or her social interaction since parenting is easier if the infant is happy and easily consolable than if the infant is fussy.

An infant's ability to provide self-comfort can be assessed by observing how quickly the infant habituates to light or the sound of a bell, how quickly the infant moves from fussing to a quiet state when aroused from sleep, or how the infant reacts to touch. A wellness diagnosis for the infant who is able to provide self-comfort might be

~ *Progressive self-comforting behavior*

CASE STUDY

To help the reader understand how wellness nursing diagnoses are used with the normal childbearing family, the following case study of a postpartum woman is presented.

B.C. is a 33-year-old woman who has been married for 10 years, has a 7-year-old son, and works outside the home. Both she and her husband are white-collar workers, own their own home, and are involved in professional and community activities. B.C. is 1 week postpartum. Her pregnancy, labor, and delivery were normal and her infant girl weighed 7 pounds. Both mother and child are doing well.

B.C. describes herself as "bright, pleasant, cooperative, and logical." She has just completed a master's degree and does not plan to have any more children. She is open to new information and says, "I would love to learn anything you have to teach me about breastfeeding and infant care." Although she bottle-fed her son, B.C. decided to breastfeed this infant. B.C. has many questions about infant care, and in particular, the care of a baby girl.

B.C. reads widely about infant care and asks many questions of her friends who have children, the nurse, and other health care professionals. Although she is comfortable holding her baby, recognizes when the baby is hungry, and demonstrates attachment behaviors, she recognizes that infant care practices have changed somewhat in 7 years and she wants to be sure she is giving her baby the best care possible.

B.C. is able to breastfeed her infant in one position. The infant latches on well and is gaining weight. B.C. recognizes that breastfeeding has increased her nutritional requirements and has adapted her diet to meet these needs.

From this information, one can see that B.C. is progressing well in her ability to care for the new baby as well as in learning how to breastfeed. Examples of wellness nursing diagnoses for this woman would be *increasing confidence in infant care skills* and *beginning establishment of breastfeeding.*

Client-centered goals for B.C. would be (1) confidence in infant care skills and (2) establishment of breastfeeding. Nursing interventions would include reinforcing B.C.'s ability to care for her infant, providing information about infant care as needed, and con firming the information that B.C. has acquired. Interventions related to the goal of establishment of breastfeeding would include information about ways to position the infant, how to recognize infant cues of satiety, and positive reinforcement of B.C.'s efforts to breastfeed. Information about resources such as La Leche League or books/pamphlets that provide breastfeeding information would also be helpful. Discussion of the pros and cons of continuing to breastfeed upon return to work would help B.C. decide what she wants to do when that time comes.

SUMMARY

Using the developmental tasks of the childbearing year, examples of wellness nursing diagnoses for the childbearing family have been given. These examples are not meant to be all-inclusive, but are presented to stimulate interest in the use of wellness nursing diagnoses, rather than problem-oriented ones, for healthy pregnant women and their families. Use of these diagnoses will provide direction for nursing care to the healthy pregnant woman and will also facilitate communication among health care providers about the care that is given. Both of these purposes will improve the quality of nursing care given to pregnant women and their families.

To further the reader's understanding of wellness nursing diagnoses, Table 4.1 (see overleaf) presents selected client behaviors and nursing interventions appropriate for each wellness nursing diagnosis discussed in this chapter.

References

Colman, L.L., and Colman, A.D. (1991). *Pregnancy: The Psychological Experience*. New York: The Noonday Press.

May, K.A. (1982). Three phases of father involvement in pregnancy. *Nursing Research, 31,* 337–342.

Mercer R.T. (1985). The process of maternal role attainment over the first year. *Nursing Research, 34*, 198–204.

Nursing Diagnoses: Definitions and Classifications 1995–1996 (1994). Philadelphia: North American Nursing Diagnosis Association.

Rubin, R. (1967). Attainment of the maternal role. Part I. Processes. *Nursing Research, 16*, 237–245.

Walker, L.O. (1992). *Parent–Infant Nursing Science: Paradigms, Phenomena, Methods.* Philadelphia: Davis.

Table 4.1. Relationships Among Selected Wellness Nursing Diagnoses, Behaviors, and Interventions: The Childbearing Family

Wellness Nursing Diagnosis	Childbearing Family Behaviors	Nursing Interventions
Beginning acceptance of reality of pregnancy**	Seeks early prenatal care	Explore feelings of ambiguity
	States she is pregnant	Reassure feelings of ambiguity are normal
	Describes ambiguity about pregnancy	Reinforce early prenatal care
	Modifies smoking or drinking habits to accommodate pregnancy	
Seeking early prenatal care*	Compares resources for provision of prenatal care	Provide information about resources for prenatal care
	Makes appointment with health care provider	Reinforce importance of early prenatal care
		Answer questions about pregnancy
		Provide information about physical changes during pregnancy

*Increasing joy about being pregnant****	Expresses feelings of joy	Reinforce feelings of joy and excitement
	Talks to others about pregnancy	Provide information regarding resources for prenatal classes, books, etc., about pregnancy
	Starts planning for coming infant	Support early planning
*Progressive incorporation of physical changes of pregnancy into lifestyle***	Describes physical changes she is experiencing	Provide information regarding physical changes as needed
	Modifies diet to reduce nausea and vomiting	Explore options for accommodating physical changes such as diet, ways to get out of chairs and/or bed as pregnancy advances
	Describes changes in body image	Answer questions as needed
	Makes changes in furniture placement, space, etc., to encourage mobility	
*Progressive acceptance of reality of the fetus****	Describes fetal movement or other indicators of fetal activity such as hiccups	Point out fetal parts during abdominal assessment

* Applies to expectant mother
** Applies to expectant mother or father
*** Can be adapted for expectant father
**** Couple
***** Father

(continued)

87

Wellness Nursing Diagnosis	Childbearing Family Behaviors	Nursing Interventions
*Progressive acceptance of reality of the fetus** (cont'd.)*	Starts looking at infant clothes	Provide way to hear fetal heart tones
		Reinforce mother's observations of fetus
		Provide information about age-appropriate fetal characteristics
*Beginning preparation of environment (nesting) for new infant**	Starts preparing a place for infant—nursery, special area, etc.	Provide information regarding clothing essentials
	Attends baby showers	Provide information about infant care classes
	Buys infant clothing, furniture, etc.	Reinforce preparation for infant
*Beginning prenatal attachment**	Talks or sings to infant	Reinforce attachment behaviors
	Uses special name for fetus	Point out fetal parts during abdominal assessment
	Pats abdomen and talks about how fetus moves	
	Starts thinking about name for baby	

*Examining relationship with own mother***	Describes ways was mothered	Explore feelings about mother's behaviors
	Accepts or rejects mother's behaviors	Provide alternatives regarding patterns of childrearing/parenting
	Plans ways to incorporate mother into care of new infant without losing own control	Assist in decision making about infant care postpartum
*Developing a working relationship directed toward mutual support during pregnancy and parenting*****	Shares feelings about pregnancy and parenthood with partner	Reinforce sharing of feelings with partner
	Recognizes partner's response to pregnancy	Provide information regarding prenatal classes
	Practices breathing and relaxation techniques with partner	Reinforce practice of breathing and relaxation techniques
	Discusses alternative parenting patterns with partner	Provide information about parenting
*Recognizing family interdependence**	Includes partner in plans for dealing with pregnancy and labor	Reinforce discussion of feelings between partners

(continued)

Wellness Nursing Diagnosis	Childbearing Family Behaviors	Nursing Interventions
Recognizing family interdependence* (cont'd.)	Shares feelings about pregnancy with partner	Explore ways to provide opportunities for partner to be involved in pregnancy, labor, and infant
	Plans for upcoming infant with other children	Reinforce inclusion of other children in plans
Beginning fantasies about infant's personality**	Describes perceptions of what infant will look and act like	Explore fantasies
	May identify gender of fetus	Reassure that "fantasies" are normal
	Attributes meaning to fetal movement	
Beginning maternal–infant attachment***	Calls infant by name	Reinforce attachment behaviors
	Points out infant characteristics that are similar to other family members	Provide opportunities for infant contact and infant care
	Holds infant in *en face* position	Point out infant responses to stimuli such as light and sound
	Recognizes that infant responds to mother's (father's) voice	

90

*Resolving conflict between fantasized and actual infant***	Describe fantasies of what expected infant will be like	Describe typical infant characteristics
	Compares beliefs about average infant with own infant's behavior	Enhance knowledge of infant through physical examination, demonstration of infant reflexes, etc.
	Modifies unrealistic expectations of infant by incorporating knowledge of own infant into description of normal newborn behaviors	Reinforce realistic expectations of infant
*Beginning attainment of maternal role****	Observes role models for mothering behaviors	Discuss patterns of mothering
	Seeks opportunities to practice infant care	Explore and/or provide opportunities for practice in child care
	Selects mothering behaviors she wishes to use in mothering infant	Reinforce practice of child care if needed
	Fantasizes about type of mother she wants to be	
*Integrating fantasy role with actual mothering role****	Describes what she believes "ideal" mother is like	Explore expectations of what she believes mothering to be like

91

(continued)

Wellness Nursing Diagnosis	Childbearing Family Behaviors	Nursing Interventions
Integrating fantasy role with actual mothering role*** (cont'd.)	Revises expectations of mothering role to accommodate her particular infant's behaviors	Reinforce realistic expectations
		Clarify misconceptions or unrealistic expectations
Progressive preparation for labor*	Explores alternative methods of preparation for labor	Provide information about alternative methods of preparation
	Attends preparation for childbirth classes	Reinforce attendance at classes
	Selects particular method of preparation and practices breathing and relaxation techniques	Observe practice of breathing and relaxation techniques and clarify any misconceptions or errors
	Reads books about labor	
Creating a labor plan to communicate personal desires for labor experience*	States preferences for labor experience such as amount and type of analgesia/anesthesia, contact with infant, episiotomy, breathing techniques, etc.	Explore realistic alternatives for labor experience
		Reinforce decision making
	Prioritizes preferences for labor experience	Communicate client preferences to other health care professionals as appropriate
	Communicates wishes to health care	

92

	provider	
Maintaining control during labor*	Breathes through contractions	Coach in breathing techniques during contractions
	Relaxes between contractions	Encourage relaxation between contractions
	Able to follow directions during contractions	Provide alternative methods of pain management if selected ones are ineffective
	Works well with partner during contractions	
Acquiring role of labor coach*****	Describes role he wishes to play during labor	Explore preferences for participation in labor experience
	Discusses wishes with partner	Explore role expectations with both partners
	Attends prepared childbirth classes	
	Practices breathing and relaxation techniques with partner	Reinforce practice of breathing and relaxation techniques
Beginning establishment of breastfeeding*	Helps infant latch on to breast	Clarify any misconceptions about breastfeeding

(continued)

Wellness Nursing Diagnosis	Childbearing Family Behaviors	Nursing Interventions
Beginning establishment of breastfeeding (cont'd.)	Demonstrates several positions of holding infant during feeding	Reinforce ability to breastfeed
	Recognizes when infant swallows	Provide additional information regarding positioning, signs that infant is satisfied, etc.
	Demonstrates ability to massage breast and express milk/colostrum	
*Increasing confidence in infant care skills***	Feeds, diapers, and bathes infant	Point out additional infant cues that reinforce parent's behavior
	Notices infant cues of hunger, distress, satisfaction	Reinforce ability to give care
	Modifies infant care skills to meet individual infant needs	
	Describes feelings of confidence	
*Beginning integration of the infant into the family***	Provides opportunities for siblings to hold infant	Explore feelings about allowing other family members to provide infant care
	Points out infant characteristics to siblings that are similar to their own	Discuss ways to involve family members in infant care

	Discuss ways to reduce sibling rivalry
	Encourages partner to help in infant care
	Plans infant care at times when other family members can help
Beginning adjustment to multiple roles*	
Recognizes conflict between roles	Discuss conflict between roles
Sets priorities related to each role	Suggest alternative ways to meet obligations of multiple roles
Accepts help from family members in order to obtain rest	Reinforce decisions to obtain adequate rest
(Neonate)	
Adequate oxygen exchange	
Pink body and extremities	Position to allow for breathing easily
No chest retraction	Remove any environmental obstacles/obstructions
Respirations 30–60 breaths/minute	
Maintenance of thermoregulation	
Temperature within normal limits (97.7°–99.5°F)	Place infant on mother's abdomen skin-to-skin after delivery
	Uncover only one part of infant at a time when assessing

95

(continued)

Wellness Nursing Diagnosis	Childbearing Family Behaviors	Nursing Interventions
Maintenance of thermoregulation (cont'd.)		Place infant on padded surface
Adequate nutritional intake	"Latches on" to breast	Help mother and infant learn to breastfeed if applicable
	Has well-developed swallowing and sucking reflexes	Show mother ways to determine that infant is swallowing
	Suckles on bottle or breast at regular intervals	Discuss feeding techniques with mother
	Well hydrated	
Progressive transition to extrauterine life	Maintains body temperature within normal limits	Provide adequate clothing
	Habituates to normal sounds	Explain normal range of infant behavior to caregiver
	Exhibits various sleep stages ranging from sleep to wakeful states	Demonstrate infant's ability to habituate to stimuli to caregiver
	Pink body and extremities	
Progressive synchrony with mother	Responds to mother's voice	Point out synchronous behavior to caregiver

	Initiates and breaks off interaction with caregiver	Explain infant's ability to initiate and terminate interaction
	Moves in rhythm to mother's voice	Help caregiver become attuned to infant's behavior
Beginning to elicit caretaking behaviors	Responds to caregiver's voice (especially mother) by turning head toward sound	Point out infant's response to caregiver
	Establishes eye contact with caregiver	Provide positive reinforcement to caregiver for child care activities
		Discuss realistic expectations for infant behavior
Progressive self-comforting behavior	After several stimuli, no longer responds to startle reflex	Explain and demonstrate infant's ability to provide self-comfort
	Calms self after startle	Discuss normal range of behavior for infant

5
~

Wellness Nursing Diagnoses for Infants

Although pediatric nurses work with ill infants in acute care settings, they also have many opportunities to care for well infants. The opportunities for focusing on wellness are increasing as health care delivery shifts to include health promotion as well as prevention and treatment of disease.

One of the settings in which healthy babies receive care is the well child clinic. Even when caring for hospitalized children, pediatric nurses emphasize attainment of developmental tasks regardless of the illness and strive to prevent regression in these tasks, thus supporting wellness behaviors. For the purposes of this chapter, infancy is defined as from birth to 1 year of life.

Complete assessment of the infant and young child includes assessment of caregivers and the environment in which the child is being raised. Examples of wellness nursing diagnoses related to the caregiver include:

~ *Progressive acquisition of realistic expectations of child's abilities*
~ *Providing a safe environment*
~ *Creating learning opportunities for the child*
~ *Providing adequate nutrition*

~ *Protecting child from infection by obtaining necessary immunizations*

~ Assessment of Strengths

Several areas of development become apparent when working with infants. General assessment areas include motor development, psychosocial development, cognitive development, and role learning (Wong, 1995). The type of play in which an infant participates also provides cues to social development.

Assessment of each of these areas provides data for the formation of wellness nursing diagnoses. However, all the significant behaviors associated with the various developmental tasks are not enumerated in this book. The reader may wish to refer to any pediatric textbook for further information.

A variety of factors influence an infant's development and there is wide variation in the range of normal behaviors among individuals. Physiologic changes are impacted by heredity and neuroendocrine responses. Social development is influenced by the interaction with others in one's environment and the learning opportunities provided in that environment. In infants and young children, the safety of an environment also affects their development because it determines the extent to which they are free to explore that environment and learn from it.

The nurse needs to keep these influences in mind when assessing the infant for attainment of various developmental tasks, when helping caretakers gain knowledge and experience in child care, and when modifying various environmental stimuli to facilitate normal development. As in other chapters, the nursing diagnoses presented here deal with the first part of the diagnosis (client response). The second part of the diagnosis (condition) is dependent on the contributing factors that will be identified in the particular client situation.

Motor Development

In the first year of life, infants have rapid motor development starting initially with gross movements that progress outward from the central trunk to the fingers and toes as they grow. Also during the first year, infants move from a dependent state in which they are unable to locomote to one in which they can walk. The various stages of rolling over, sitting, crawling, standing, and walking occur along a continuum of normal progression that is age specific, but is modified by a variety of environmental factors.

Assessment questions the nurse might ask of self or others include:

- How has the infant met the motor development tasks appropriate for his age?
- In what ways is the infant allowed to move freely in a safe environment?
- What is the caretaker doing to provide stimulation to help the infant develop motor skills?

To indicate that the infant has a normal pattern of motor development for the first year of life, an appropriate nursing diagnosis is

~ *Progressive development of motor skills*

Data for this type of diagnosis would indicate that the infant has age-appropriate skills and that these skills are progressively becoming more refined.

Psychosocial Development

The psychosocial developmental task most prominent in the first year of life is the development of trust (Erikson, 1963). In psychoanalytic terms, most activities are oral and provide a way of getting to know the world, getting one's needs met, and obtaining pleasure. The caregiver relationship is central to the recognition that one's needs will be met, and as a whole, the infant is unable to differentiate himself from the caregiver.

Behaviors in the latter half of the first year of life that would indicate progressive development of trust include exploring the environment freely with limited fear, placing objects in the mouth as the infant finds them in the environment, responding to various colors and textures with squeals of delight or grimaces of dislike, and gradual acceptance of delayed gratification. Toward the end of the first year, the child will have overcome some of the stranger anxiety present at 4–8 months.

Although a wide variety of behaviors are exhibited during the first year, they progress through a normal sequence. When assessing psychosocial development, the nurse might consider the following questions:

- Does the infant explore the environment without fear? If so, how?
- What are the infant's responses to new toys or persons in the environment?
- How quickly does the infant respond to changes in the environment?

A wellness diagnosis related to psychosocial development could be

~ *Beginning sense of trust*

Cognitive Development

The infant learns through interaction with the environment and those who care for him. Such learning is carried out through the senses of taste, smell, touch, sight, and hearing. Learning occurs primarily through trial and error and progresses from reflex activity to imitative behaviors. As children approach the second year, they are able to differentiate themselves from the environment. A high level of curiosity exists.

Wellness nursing diagnoses related to cognitive development during the first year of life could center on one or more of the following themes: change from reflex activity to association between a stimulus and a response; imitative acts that produce pleasure in the infant; object permanence where the infant can remember an object even if it is no longer in sight; and beginning association of symbols (verbal sounds/language) with objects or events.

Behaviors that would indicate recognition of event sequencing include anticipation of being fed upon seeing mother or caregiver, association of a bottle or breast with feeding before it is placed in one's mouth, or walking to the door when one's coat is put on. Performance of imitative acts becomes evident when the child enters into games such as peek-a-boo or mimics the facial expression of others. The beginning of object permanence is demonstrated when the child continues to look for a toy after it has been removed. Beginning acquisition of verbal skills occurs when syllables such as ma-ma or da-da are spoken when the adult enters the room.

Assessment questions could include:

- What kinds of associations does the infant make with objects in the environment?
- Does the infant imitate sounds and enjoy repetitive activities such as peek-a-boo?
- Does the infant remember where an object is even if it can no longer be seen?
- What kinds of verbal sounds does the infant make and are they associated with particular persons or objects?

Examples of wellness nursing diagnoses include:

- ~ Beginning recognition of event sequencing
- ~ Performing imitative acts
- ~ Beginning recognition of object permanence
- ~ Beginning acquisition of verbal skills

Role Learning

The infant is unaware of any perspective other than his own. All activity is egocentric. Socialization throughout the year progresses from smiling at caretakers to actively seeking to be held. Interest in pleasing the caretaker, especially the mother, becomes evident toward the end of the first year of life. Some assessment questions might include:

- Does the infant smile?
- How does the infant respond to caregivers?
- In what ways does the infant try to please parents or caregivers?
- Does the infant cuddle or seek attention through touch? At what times?

A wellness nursing diagnosis would be

~ *Progressive interaction with family members*

Play

Infants interact with others and respond to them through play. Such games as pat-a-cake and peek-a-boo create enthusiasm and children learn that adults gain pleasure when they respond positively. Additionally, one can see the pleasure in a child's face when repeating a skill that has been learned. These skills may include shaking a rattle, banging an object against a solid surface to hear the noise, or continuously turning the handle of a jack-in-the-box.

Questions for assessment of play might include:

- What kinds of games does the infant enjoy?
- How does the infant display curiosity about new things?
- How pleased is the infant with new activities?
- What kinds of repetitive activities does the infant display?

This wellness nursing diagnosis would be useful:

~ *Beginning expressions of pleasure associated with repetitive activities*

CASE STUDY

To illustrate the use of wellness nursing diagnoses in infants, the following case study is presented.

J.W. is a 9-month-old infant who has two siblings. He is within normal height and weight limits for his age. J.W. enjoys playing pat-a-cake with his older brother and one sees an expression of joy on his face when his brother comes into the room. He has just learned to walk and enjoys exploring all corners of a room looking for toys or just feeling the sofa or curtains. When J.W. sees adults who have familiar faces, he grins and holds out his hands to be picked up. Although still a little wary of strange adults, he is becoming more comfortable with strangers as long as his mother is close at hand.

Some wellness nursing diagnoses for J.W. include *progressive development of motor skills, beginning sense of trust,* and *beginning expressions of pleasure associated with repetitive activities.*

Goals for J.W. would be (a) continued acquisition of skills and (b) progressive attainment of the sense of trust. Some nursing interventions with J.W.'s parents would include teaching about normal growth and development, discussion of how to provide a safe environment in which J.W. can continue to explore, and discussion of age-appropriate toys and activities that will encourage curiosity and development of gross and fine motor skills.

SUMMARY

The examples of wellness nursing diagnoses for infants, based on developmental tasks, presented in this chapter represent only a small portion of those that might be developed for the first year of life. Considering the multiple changes occurring during that time, the possibilities for these nursing diagnoses are endless. The author hopes that those experienced in working with infants will see this chapter as a framework for developing these types of diagnoses and encourages them to continue this work.

To further the reader's understanding of the use of wellness nursing diagnoses with infants, Table 5.1 (see overleaf) illustrates the relationships among the diagnoses discussed in this chapter, examples of behaviors appropriate to the diagnoses, and examples of nursing interventions.

References

Erikson, E.H. (1963). *Childhood and Society* (2nd ed.). New York: Norton.

Wong, D. (1995). *Whaley and Wong's Nursing Care of Infants and Children* (5th ed.). St. Louis: Mosby–Year Book.

Table 5.1. Relationships Among Selected Wellness Nursing Diagnoses, Behaviors, and Interventions: Infants

Wellness Nursing Diagnosis	Infant Behaviors	Nursing Interventions
Progressive development of motor skills	Age-specific motor skills are within normal limits and progress along a continuum: lying flat, lifting chin, rolling over, sitting, crawling, pulling self up, standing, etc.	Help caregiver establish realistic expectations for infant
		Explain normal progression of motor skills to caregiver and help prepare for next skill to be developed
		Point out infant's progress to caregiver if necessary
Beginning sense of trust	Explores environment freely	Explain necessity of developing a sense of trust
	Places new objects in mouth	Discuss creation of a safe environment
	Reaches out to others	Discuss ways to provide different stimuli for infant (colors, textures, sounds)
Beginning recognition of event sequencing	Recognizes familiar objects and faces	Discuss normal progression of behaviors with caregiver

	Shows excitement when coat is put on or bottle is held up	Reinforce caretaking activities that promote growth and development
	Associates sounds with objects	
Performance of imitative acts	Mimics facial expressions of others	Encourage caregiver to play games with infant
	Plays pat-a-cake or peek-a-boo	Discuss normal progression of behaviors
	Engages in repetitive behaviors such as banging a object against a solid surface	Reinforce caregiver's activities that promote growth and development
	Imitates sounds	Discuss normal range of behaviors
Beginning recognition of object permanence	Looks for toy after it has been removed	Discuss implications of object permanence—will have to find new ways to distract infant if necessary
	Looks for mother after she has left the room	
Beginning acquisition of verbal skills	Uses nonsense syllables	Discuss normal progression of vocal skills
	Makes sounds to gain attention	Point out specific behaviors to caregiver

(continued)

Wellness Nursing Diagnosis	Infant Behaviors	Nursing Interventions
Beginning acquisition of verbal skills (cont'd.)	Makes sounds to denote particular objects	Clarify expectations caregiver has for infant
	Understands the word *no*	
Progressive interaction with family members	Smiles at family members	Point out infant's interactive behaviors
	Recognizes family members when they enter field of vision	Discuss normal progression of behaviors
	Reaches out for family members—grasps hands	
	Plays games with family members	
Beginning expressions of pleasure associated with repetitive activities	Smiles while shakes rattle or bangs object on floor	Encourage interaction with infant
	Laughs, squeals at particular sounds or toys	Discuss provision of age-appropriate toys
	Plays peek-a-boo with enthusiasm	Discuss ways to encourage child's enthusiasm

6
~

Wellness Nursing Diagnoses for Toddlers and Preschool Children

Although pediatric nurses work with ill children in acute care settings, they also work with healthy children who receive care in day care centers and preschools. Even when caring for hospitalized children, pediatric nurses recognize that these children have strengths. Fostering these strengths helps the child continue to progress through the appropriate developmental tasks.

Major areas of health promotion related to the young child deal with supplying adequate nutrition, immunizing against various contagious diseases, providing a safe environment, and fostering feelings of security, love, and worth. The child is dependent on the caregiver to provide the necessary components to maintain adequate physical growth and development. In addition, the caregiver promotes interactions conducive to the child's psychosocial growth and development, resulting in formation of a separate identity that recognizes the worth of both the self and others. See Chapter 5 for wellness nursing diagnoses related to the caregiver.

∼ *Assessment of Strengths*

As in Chapter 5, general assessment areas will include motor development, psychosocial development, cognitive development, role learning and play. Assessment of each of these areas provides data for the formation of wellness nursing diagnoses. As in Chapter 5, some specific age-appropriate data and nursing diagnoses will be provided, although all the significant behaviors associated with the various developmental tasks are not listed.

A variety of factors influence a toddler and preschool child's development. Provision of a safe environment, opportunities to acquire new experiences that will enhance motor skills, and increased social interaction all contribute to the growth and development of this group of children. Assessment data can be obtained from observation of the child, questioning the caretaker, and evaluation of the environment in which the child lives and/or plays.

As in other chapters, the nursing diagnoses presented here deal with the first part of the diagnosis (client response). The second part of the diagnosis (condition) is dependent on the contributing factors that will be identified in the particular client situation.

Motor Development

This period is one of intense activity and continuous exploration of the world. Once the fundamental gross motor activities of sitting, standing, and walking are mastered, the child progresses to more active movements including running, jumping, throwing, and catching. As the child continues development of gross motor activity, fine motor coordination is acquired or refined as well.

Completion of jigsaw puzzles, putting various shaped blocks in the appropriate shaped hole, scribbling with crayons, and turning the pages of a book while someone reads a story are all examples of use of fine motor skills. Assessment questions that the nurse might ask herself or others include:

- What kind of fine motor activities does the child exhibit?
- What toys does the child have that facilitate fine motor activities?
- What gross motor activities has the child learned and is there progression in the complexity of these activities?

Although the specific behaviors vary depending on the age of the child, a wellness diagnosis that could be used at any time with this age group would be

~ *Progressive refining of motor skills*

Psychosocial Development

Psychoanalytic theory states that the anal stage of psychosexual development is prominent during ages 1 to 3, and children learn to control their ability to withhold or expel. The developmental task of autonomy focuses on the 1- to 3-year-old and encompasses the notion of control of self and one's environment (Erikson, 1963). A basic conflict between the need for independence and a wish to remain dependent occurs during this time.

The physical development that promotes and allows toilet training is also a metaphor for the social and cognitive development that simultaneously occurs. Thus, the child learns to "hold on" and "let go" in many areas of life. As children learn to express their will, the word *no* becomes prominent in their vocabulary. Parents may become exasperated at the negativism present in the toddler's life. To retain some security during this time of "letting go," the child engages in ritualistic behavior such as repetitive chants, performing tasks in the same way, or playing with particular toys. Assessment questions might include:

- Has the child started potty training and how well is the child progressing?
- What kinds of ritualistic behavior does the child exhibit?
- Does the child display autonomous behaviors such as saying "no" or running away from the caregiver when called?

A wellness nursing diagnosis that would reflect the activities listed above would be

~ *Beginning sense of autonomy*

According to psychoanalytic theory, the 3- to 6-year-old moves into the phallic stage with beginning interest in sexual differences culminating in identification with the same-sex parent. According to Erikson (1963), the psychosocial task for the preschooler is developing a sense of initiative. During this phase, the child explores the world to the utmost. The imagination becomes active and plays a large role in the child's life. In addition, the child learns how to gain satisfaction without impinging on the rights of others. A conscience comes into being and learning right from wrong is a major task. Most learning still comes from experiences with parents and family members. Some assessment questions that the nurse might use include:

- How does the child demonstrate knowledge of right from wrong?
- How does the child use imagination? Does he or she have an imaginary playmate? Can the child describe the things he or she draws?
- Can the child play alone for an extended period of time?

A wellness nursing diagnosis would be

~ *Beginning sense of initiative*

Cognitive Development

Piaget (1975) describes the cognitive development for the child 2 to 7 years of age as the preoperational phase. The term *operations* describes the ability to manipulate objects logically in relation to each other. This phase is separated into two stages: preconceptual (ages 2–4) and intuitive thought (ages 4–7). Children in the preconceptual stage are egocentric and interpret objects and the world in light of their own experience. They can deal only with concrete objects, neglecting to go beyond the observable. Toward the end of the phase, ability to make simple connections between ideas begins and intuitive reasoning is used. However, measurement of objects is obtained only from perceptual cues and awareness of similarities among same-sized objects with varying heights or widths is not possible. Children also start to develop a social awareness that includes acknowledgment of others' viewpoints.

Language development is rapid from ages 2 to 4. Children love to hear themselves talk. Prior to age 3, most language is related to the self, such as "I want," "I do." Reasoning is related to particular objects and no amount of prodding can lead to generalizations. Sometime during the second year, the child gains an interest in "why" things work. Language continues to be egocentric until the child reaches school age.

Responses will vary depending on the child's age, but some assessment questions that might be useful include:

- What is the child's level of language development? Do most statements begin with "I"?
- How much does the child talk? Is much of it repetitive or "silly" sayings?
- How often does the child ask "why"?
- How does the child deal with the concrete, particular object?

Wellness nursing diagnoses for this age group could be

~ *Rapid increase in language skills*
~ *Preoperational thinking*

Role Learning

Role learning is minimal at this point since the child sees the world solely from a personal viewpoint. Through play, children may imitate the roles they see adults perform, but they have no concept of what the role involves. Assessment questions might include:

- What kind of role imitation does the child do?
- How does the child interact with other children in this role imitation?

An appropriate wellness nursing diagnosis would be

~ *Beginning social interaction through imitation*

Play

Fantasy and imagination predominate the play used during this period. Between the ages of 1 and 3, children participate in parallel play that involves being beside other children but not interacting with them in a social fashion. In addition, most senses are used in play activities and form a foundation on which children base their world. Use of touch, smell, vision, and hearing help children develop fine motor skills and provide sensory input about the world.

Imitation and imagination facilitate learning the identities modeled by the family as the child practices what is seen in everyday life. Using toys that are similar to items adults use, such as toy kitchens, trucks, and lawn mowers, facilitate this process. Play becomes the work of the child as he or she seeks to understand the world. Assessment questions could include:

- What senses are used when the child plays? Does the child have a variety of toys to stimulate the senses (such as musical toys)?
- What opportunities does the child have to play with water, fingerpaints, etc.?
- In what kind of play does the child engage to encourage development of language skills?
- In what kinds of fantasies does the child engage during play?
- Does he or she play regularly with other children?
- How does the child interact with other children during play?

A wellness nursing diagnosis would be

~ *Increasing self-expression in play activities*

CASE STUDY

To illustrate the use of wellness nursing diagnoses in toddlers and preschool children, the following case study is presented.

Betty is a 3-year-old who attends preschool. Betty is a busy little girl who seldom is quiet except when asleep. She chatters constantly to herself and any one who will listen to her, often reciting repetitive nonsense that she makes up as she goes along. Her parents report that she has learned many new words in the past few months.

Betty is content to play beside another child, but makes little effort to include that child in her play. She frequently asks "why" things happen or how things work. In addition, she plays with toys that allow her to imitate her mother doing housework.

Wellness nursing diagnoses for Betty include *beginning sense of initiative, rapid increase in language skills,* and *beginning social interaction through imitation.* Goals for Betty would include (a) continued development of sense of initiative, (b) continued language development, and (c) increased social interaction. Interventions could include provision of toys that facilitate language development and fantasy play and discussion of normal growth and development with caregivers.

SUMMARY

Examples of wellness nursing diagnoses for toddlers and preschool children have been presented in this chapter. Considering the multiple physical, psychological, social, and spiritual changes that occur during these years, there are many other possibilities for nursing diagnoses. The author hopes that those nurses experienced in working with toddlers and preschool children will continue to develop wellness diagnoses for this age group.

To further the reader's understanding of the use of wellness nursing diagnoses with toddlers and preschool children, Table 6.1 (see overleaf) illustrates the relationships among the diagnoses discussed in this chapter, examples of behaviors appropriate to the diagnoses, and examples of nursing interventions.

References

Erikson, E.H. (1963). *Childhood and Society*, 2nd ed. New York: Norton.

Piaget, J. (1975). *The Construction of Reality in the Child*. New York: Ballentine Books.

Table 6.1. Relationships Among Selected Wellness Nursing Diagnoses, Behaviors, and Interventions: Toddlers and Preschool Children

Wellness Nursing Diagnosis	Toddler and Preschool Child Behaviors	Nursing Interventions
Progressive refining of motor skills	Continuous use of motor skills such as walking and early stages of running, catching, throwing	Discuss normal progression with caregiver
		Discuss ways to provide a safe environment now that child is more active
	Fine motor skills come into use such as putting together a jigsaw puzzle, scribbling with crayons, etc.	Discuss age-appropriate toys and activities that encourage development and refinement of gross and fine motor skills
Beginning sense of autonomy	Begins potty training	Explain developmental tasks and reasons for why behavior is occurring
	Uses word no indiscriminately	Discuss ways to discipline and set limits
	Learns many ways of "holding on" and "letting go" such as spitting, throwing, holding on tightly, dropping, etc.	Listen to caregiver's frustration and help problem solve how to deal with negative child

(continued)

117

Wellness Nursing Diagnosis	Toddler and Preschool Child Behaviors	Nursing Interventions
Beginning sense of autonomy (*cont'd.*)	Engages caretaker in dropping and picking up games	
	Engages in ritualistic behavior—things must be done in specific way, uses repetitive chants, etc.	
Beginning sense of initiative	Explores world widely and with much enthusiasm	Explain normal developmental tasks
		Discuss ways to provide safe environment during this time of wide exploration
	Uses imagination widely in play	Discuss age-appropriate toys with caregiver
	Starts differentiating right from wrong	
Rapid increase in language skills	Enjoys hearing self talk	Encourage child to talk
	Increase in vocabulary	Explain to parent that it may take time to understand what the child is saying; that what children say is a reflection of what they think about themselves
	Starts putting sentences together	
	Constantly asks "why"	
	Interaction is egocentric	

Preoperational thinking	Deals with one idea at a time	Discuss child's perceptual ability with caregiver
	Sees things concretely—cannot go beyond observable	If child is a finicky eater, discuss ways to manipulate amounts of food or liquid so that child will more readily eat them
	Bases perceptual judgment on what is seen, not on logical deduction	
Beginning social interaction through imitation	Pretends to cook, sweep floor, drive car, etc.	Discuss age-appropriate toys with caregiver
	May have imaginary playmate	Explain role of imaginary playmates to caregiver
	Beginning ability to share toys	
Increasing self-expression in play activities	Uses toys that are replicas of adult objects to act out mother's or father's role (e.g., iron, stove, lawn mower, etc.)	Discuss age-appropriate toys with caregiver
	Creates things from construction paper, clay, or other toys that allow creativity	Reinforce creative activity of child with both child and caregiver
		Explore ways to allow creativity with caregiver

7
~

Wellness Nursing Diagnoses for School-Age Children

Nurses care for school-age children in hospitals, schools, and clinics. These children demonstrate strengths even when hospitalized. Assessment of the child, family, and environment will help the nurse identify areas of strength that can be used to help the child cope with illness or progress through age-appropriate developmental tasks.

~ Assessment of Strengths

The same general assessment areas described in Chapters 5 and 6 will be considered in this chapter, including motor development, psychosocial development, cognitive development, and role learning. As previously recognized, the type of play in which a child participates also provides cues to social development.

Assessment of each of these areas provides the basis for wellness nursing diagnoses. In this chapter, some specific age-appropriate data and nursing diagnoses will be provided, although all the significant behaviors associated with the various developmental tasks are not presented.

As in other chapters, the nursing diagnoses presented here deal with the first part of the diagnosis (client response). The second part of the diagnosis (condition) is dependent on the contributing factors that will be identified in the particular client situation.

Motor Development

Motor development at this age expands to learning how to play various sports and emphasizes skill development. Motor activity becomes more refined, more automatic, and smoother than in the early years. The child is less clumsy, possesses the coordination necessary for participation in team sports, and is able, in most instances, to accommodate physical activity to growth spurts. The child may take part in intramural sports activities.

Eye–hand coordination improves and becomes more refined during this period. Those children who are not particularly athletic, or who not enjoy sports, may develop other hobbies that promote fine motor activity such as using computers, or building model airplanes, trains, and the like. Assessment questions related to motor development might include the following:

- What types of activities does the child participate in that require large muscle groups?
- How does the child feel about participating in sports?
- Does the child participate in any activities that require fine eye–hand coordination? How capable is the child of carrying out these activities?

A wellness nursing diagnosis would be

~ *Continuing refinement of motor skills*

Psychosocial Development

In Freudian terms, this period of psychosexual development is described as the latent period. Energies are channeled into learning particular skills, active play, and knowledge acquisition. Erikson (1963) describes this as a time for development of industry. At this age, the child learns to work with others, social relationships become prominent, and a sense of competition occurs. Rules are learned and the child wants and develops a sense of accomplishment. Much learning occurs through teachers and peers rather than primarily through the family. Assessment questions that nurses might ask of themselves, the child, or the child's family include:

- How is the child doing in school?
- How does the child act in competitive situations?
- Does the child work in groups? If so, how does he or she participate—actively, or as a passive member?
- What kind of social relationships does the child have?
- From where does the child derive pleasure?
- In what areas does the child feel successful?

Some wellness nursing diagnoses for psychosocial development in this age group are

- ~ *Beginning sense of industry*
- ~ *Beginning recognition of personal competence*
- ~ *Eagerness to engage in social activities*
- ~ *Joy and satisfaction with personal accomplishments*

Cognitive Development

Piaget (1975) describes this stage as a time of concrete operations. Thought processes become increasingly complex and logical. The child is able to sort and organize facts. Problem solving is still concrete and reflects the child's own experience. However, thought becomes less self-centered and the child is able to consider the viewpoints of others. The nurse might use the following questions for assessment:

- What kind of problem solving is the child able to do?
- How does the child use facts to describe an event?
- Is the child able to consider the viewpoints of others when describing a conflict?
- What kind of school activities does the child engage in and what kind of grades does he or she receive?

Wellness diagnoses include:

~ *Increasing ability for complex thinking*
~ *Successful achievement in school*

Role Learning

The process of learning to take on a role begins at this age. In the early years (6–8), children learn there are perspectives other than their own. However, they are still unable to imagine how others think or how they will react. In the middle years (8–10), children are able to recognize that various viewpoints may conflict and are able to consider another's point of view. In the later years (10–12), children can consider two viewpoints simultaneously and can predict the reactions of others to a particular viewpoint. The following assessment questions might be used:

- How willing is the child to consider other viewpoints?
- How many viewpoints can the child consider at the same time?
- What kind of role behaviors does the child exhibit?

A wellness nursing diagnosis would be

~ *Increasing ability to consider alternative viewpoints*

Play

Play is often centered around competitive sports and games. Indeed, play becomes the event around which social interaction is accomplished. The child enjoys making new friends, participates in group activities such as Scouts or 4-H club meetings, and often plays in small cohesive same-sex groups. Assessment questions could be:

- In what kind of group activities does the child engage?
- How well does the child function in a group?
- How easily does the child make friends?
- Who are the child's friends and what importance do they play in his or her life?

Wellness diagnoses include

> ~ *Beginning cooperative play*
> ~ *Increasing social interaction*

~ *Adaptation to Life Events*

Change is ubiquitous in everyone's life. Although most of the following life events are not unique to the school-age child, inclusion of this material in the chapter on the school-age child seems appropriate.

Life-event changes that require adaptation for the child may occur when parents move, necessitating making new friends, negotiating a new school system, or settling into a new home. Changes in family structure such as parental divorce or remarriage are common in today's culture. Assessment of the child's ability to cope with these changes is a major task of the nurse. If any of these life-event changes occur, the nurse might consider the following assessment questions:

- What kinds of things does the child do to retain old friends?
- What efforts does the child exert to make new friends?
- How successful is the child in school?
- Has the child made changes in his or her room to reflect interests and hobbies?
- What kind of interactions does the child have with new family members?
- How accepting is the child of new family members?

Examples of wellness nursing diagnoses related to these lifestyle changes include

> ~ *Beginning adaptation to new school*
> ~ *Incorporating new family members into personal social system*

Care of the hospitalized child includes efforts to reduce regression in developmental tasks as much as possible. Children with acute or chronic illnesses may experience hospitalization or have encounters with a variety of health care providers. The courage of the child with cancer who has to undergo chemotherapy, body image changes, and painful procedures has been documented by Hasse (1987). Likewise, the child who is hospitalized has to conquer fear of needles, fear of strangers, and feelings of isolation and loneliness. Assessment questions for use in these events might include:

- What kinds of adaptation has the child made to chronic illness?
- How does the child explain the illness to friends?
- How does the child react to procedures, needle sticks, and the like?
- How does the child respond to the presence of health care professionals?

Some wellness diagnoses related to these events are

~ *Beginning adaptation to chronic illness*
~ *Conquering fears of hospitalization*
~ *Incorporating physical changes into lifestyle*

CASE STUDY

To illustrate the use of wellness nursing diagnoses in the school-age child, the following case study is presented.

Joey is an 9-year-old fourth-grader with two siblings. Because of a plant closing, the family recently moved to a larger community where Joey's father, an assembly-line worker, could continue employment.

Joey is in good physical health. He is active in sports. He admires his soccer coach and expresses the desire "to be like him." Joey collects baseball cards and occasionally puts a model airplane together with the help of his father. He enjoys school and has always been a good student, making A's and B's in his classes. He likes working in groups at school but often wants to talk more than work. He has insisted on getting large athletic shirts with the state university emblem on them because "all of the boys" in his new school wear them. Although new to the school, he has actively sought out new friends. He misses his friends from his previous home, but he states that "the guys here like me" and "I think I will get to play halfback on our soccer team here like I did before."

Examples of wellness nursing diagnoses that would be appropriate for Joey include *beginning adaptation to new school, progressive sense of industry,* and *successful achievement in school.* Goals for Joey would be (a) adaptation to new school, (b) attainment of sense of industry, and (c) continued success in school.

Nursing interventions might include positive reinforcement for efforts to adapt to the new school environment, encouragement to continue to make new friends, exploration of personal interests, and praise for scholastic achievement and completion of school tasks.

SUMMARY

The examples of wellness nursing diagnoses for school-age children presented in this chapter represent only a small portion of those that might be developed using the developmental tasks of this age group. The author hopes that those nurses experienced in working with school-age children will see this chapter as a framework for developing wellness diagnoses and encourages them to continue this work.

To further the reader's understanding of the use of wellness nursing diagnoses with school-age children, Tables 7.1 and 7.2 (see overleaf) illustrate the relationships among the diagnoses discussed in this chapter, examples of behaviors appropriate to the diagnoses, and examples of nursing interventions.

References

Erikson, E.H. (1963). *Childhood and Society,* 2nd ed. New York: Norton.

Hasse, J.E. (1987). Components of courage in chronically ill adolescents: A phenomenological study. *Advances in Nursing Science*, 9(2), 64–80.

Piaget, J. (1975). *The Construction of Reality in the Child*. New York: Ballentine Books.

Table 7.1. Relationships Among Selected Wellness Nursing Diagnoses, Behaviors, and Interventions: School-Age Children

Wellness Nursing Diagnosis	School-Age Child Behaviors	Nursing Interventions
Continuing refinement of motor skills	Eye–hand coordination improves over time	Reinforce child's physical activity
	Enjoys physical activity such as running, jumping, climbing, etc.	Provide opportunities for child to increase eye–hand coordination
	Learns physical skills such as riding bicycle, skating, etc.	Discuss age-appropriate activities with caregiver and/or child
Beginning sense of industry	Interested in learning new skills	Reinforce success with child and/or caregiver
	Continues until task is completed	Discuss potential activities and ways to provide opportunities to participate in such activities with child and caregiver
	Wishes to be successful in school, games, etc.	
	Seeks peer approval	
Beginning recognition of personal competence	Engaging in self-evaluation	Encourage child to perform realistic self-evaluation
	States what he or she can do well	Reinforce child's pride
		Discuss ways to provide opportunities for

	Expresses pride in ability	continued success with child and caregiver
Eagerness to engage in social activities	Participates in group activities	Encourage child to continue social interaction
	Seeks new friendships	Help child gain new perspectives by discussing child's and other's viewpoints with him or her
	Values peer's opinions	
	Seeks peer approval	Reinforce child's satisfaction
Joy and satisfaction with personal accomplishments	Expresses joy in activities	Discuss ways to find opportunities for success with child and caregiver
	Describes personal accomplishments	
	Masters new skills	Encourage child's attempts to learn new skills
Increasing ability for complex thinking	Beginning to describe relationships between objects	Provide child with age-appropriate toys and games that encourage complex thinking
	Recognition that change in shape does not cause change in volume	Reinforce child's complex thinking
		Explore consequences of behavior with child

(continued)

Wellness Nursing Diagnosis	School-Age Child Behaviors	Nursing Interventions
Increasing ability for complex thinking (cont'd.)	Ability to think through consequences of actions	and encourage caretaker to do so
Successful achievement in school	Masters content appropriate to grade level	Reinforce child's success
	Receives positive reinforcement from teachers	Provide child with learning materials appropriate to age level and ability
	Receives recognition for participation in both curricular and extracurricular activities	Discuss ways to provide extracurricular learning experiences such as trips to museums and zoo with child and caregiver
Increasing ability to consider alternative viewpoints	Able to state other's viewpoint	Reinforce child's consideration of other's viewpoints in decision making
	Recognizes that other's viewpoint may conflict with his or her own	Explore alternative actions and subsequent consequences with child
	Can predict how others will respond to his or her viewpoint	
Beginning cooperative play	Joins group activities	Encourage child's activities with group
	Learns rules of peer group	Explore rewards child gains from group
		Discuss potential conflict with child and

	Subordinates own wishes to that of group	caregiver that might arise between child/family values and peer group values and suggest ways to resolve conflict
Increasing social interaction	Contributes to group interaction when making decisions	Encourage child's social interaction with peers/friends, etc.
	Develops intimate relationship with same-sex friend	Discuss with child ways to work with group to attain mutual goals

Table 7.2. Relationships Among Selected Wellness Nursing Diagnoses, Behaviors, and Interventions: Adaptation to Life Events

Wellness Nursing Diagnosis	School-Age Child Behaviors	Nursing Interventions
Beginning adaptation to new school	Making new friends	Explore ways to gain new friends
	Selecting extracurricular activities	Reinforce seeking new activities
	States that "it is becoming easier to be at school"	Explore what child thinks are the strengths and weaknesses of the new school
Incorporating new family members into personal social system	Includes new siblings in play activities	Provide opportunity for child to discuss feelings about the changes
	Seeks help from new parent	Reinforce acceptance of changes
	Willing to make changes in own schedule to allow visitation with other parent	Explore ways that child can continue to include new family members in activities
Beginning adaptation to chronic illness	Describes symptoms of illness	Explore ways that illness is affecting lifestyle
	Knows how to obtain help if needed	Provide information about medication, signs and symptoms of illness, etc., as needed
	Knows type and amount of medication if	

applicable	Reinforce accurate information
Recognizes when he or she needs help (such as signs and symptoms of insulin reaction)	
Conquering fears of hospitalization	Be honest with child
Describes feelings about hospitalization or acts them out in play	Comfort through physical contact as necessary
Accepts treatments	Provide opportunities for child to express feelings
Allows parent to leave for short intervals without crying	Stay with child during procedures
Begins relationship with nurses and other hospital staff	Incorporate caregiver into plan of care
	Provide opportunities for caregiver to discuss feelings
Incorporating physical changes into lifestyle	Reinforce knowledge
Child can describe physical changes	Explore ways that child can participate in school activities even if limited
Child and caregiver plan activities appropriate for child's ability and/or limitations	Discuss alternative activities

Karen M. Stolte: WELLNESS NURSING
DIAGNOSIS FOR HEALTH PROMOTION.
© 1996 Lippincott–Raven Publishers.

8
~

Wellness Nursing Diagnoses for Adolescents

Although pediatric nurses work with adolescents in acute care settings, they also have other opportunities to care for well adolescents. For example, nursing care of healthy adolescents occurs in family planning clinics, school settings, and adolescent clinics. Thus, there is a need for wellness nursing diagnoses to guide care that focuses on strengths of the adolescent client rather than prevention of potential problems when, in fact, the potential may not exist.

~ *Assessment of Strengths*

The general assessment areas of psychosocial development, cognitive development, and role learning are used in this chapter. Examples of wellness nursing diagnoses will be provided, although all the significant behaviors associated with the various developmental tasks are not specified.

As in other chapters, the nursing diagnoses presented here deal with the first part of the diagnosis (client response). The second part of the diagnosis (condition) is dependent on the contributing factors, which will be identified in the particular client situation.

Psychosocial Development

In psychoanalytic terms, the genital phase occurs during adolescence and is the major source of sexual tension. Energies are focused on relationships with old and new friends. Experiences with these relationships provide preparation for marriage. A sense of identity (Erikson, 1963) must be developed. Adolescence is a time of turmoil involving marked physical and biological changes. Struggles with self-concept and body image (how one appears to others, particularly peers) and the need to develop some plan for life contribute to this inner turmoil. The need for intimate relationships is strong and reliance on peer approval is dominant. Decisions about occupational choice also occur during this time.

Assessment questions that nurses might ask themselves, the client, or others in the client's environment include:

- How does the client feel about himself or herself?
- What kind of relationships does the adolescent have with others? Same sex? Opposite sex?
- How does the client feel about the physical changes that occurred during puberty?
- Has the adolescent begun to think about what occupation to pursue?
- Whose opinions does the client value? If these opinions are in conflict with parental authority, what does the adolescent do?

Examples of wellness nursing diagnoses related to the adolescent are

- ~ *Beginning sense of personal identity*
- ~ *Increasing interest in opposite sex*
- ~ *Incorporating secondary sex changes into body image*
- ~ *Beginning formulation of occupational goals*
- ~ *Beginning separation from family authority*

Cognitive Development

The adolescent is able to think in abstract terms. Thinking becomes more flexible and adaptable. As a result, the adolescent is able to draw conclusions from observations, make hypotheses, and test them. Piaget (1975) calls this the stage of formal operations. Assessment questions might include:

- How flexible is the adolescent? Can he or she see other viewpoints?
- What achievements has the adolescent had in school?
- Can the adolescent handle abstract concepts?
- How accurate is the adolescent when making conclusions?

Wellness nursing diagnoses related to this stage would include

~ *Increasing consideration of others' opinions*
~ *Increasing ability for abstract reasoning*

Role Learning

Awareness of the social impact of roles allows the adolescent to consider roles in light of the social order. Social mores of the peer group have a major influence on the adolescent, often resulting in fads and behavior peculiar to one particular group. Those who do not fit the social mores are excluded from the group. As a preparation for marriage, social relationships become more intimate and often change from group interactions to a relationship with one individual. Leisure interests range from those of one's same-sex peer group to those that include both sexes. Assessment questions might include:

- What kind of fads or social behaviors does the adolescent imitate from the peer group?
- What kinds of social relationships does the adolescent have? With others of the same sex? With members of the opposite sex?
- Are the majority of relationships with one member of the opposite sex, with peer groups, or with members of the same sex?
- How is leisure time spent? What hobbies does the adolescent have?

Wellness nursing diagnoses in this area include

~ *Developing potentially long-lasting relationships*

~ *Developing relationships with opposite-sex peers*
~ *Increasing personal interests and hobbies*

CASE STUDY

To illustrate the use of wellness nursing diagnoses in adolescents, the following case study is presented.

Larry is a 16-year-old who participates in the sports program of his high school. He has a small group of boys with which he socializes a great deal. However, he also has a growing interest in a female member of his class. Thus, his interest in his personal appearance has increased as has the time spent on personal hygiene. He has started dating, and he and his date sometimes double date with another couple.

Larry is well versed with computers and is interested in being a computer programmer. Much of his free time is spent reading about computers and learning different computer programs.

Wellness nursing diagnoses for Larry include *beginning sense of personal identity, increasing interest in the opposite sex,* and *beginning formulation of occupational goals.* Nursing goals would be (a) continued development of personal identity, (b) continued social development, and (c) formulation of occupational goal. Interventions directed toward these goals could include reinforcement of personal hygiene behaviors, praise for accomplishments, encouragement in dating, and discussion of occupational interests.

SUMMARY

Some questions have been presented for assessment of the adolescent related to the developmental tasks of this age group. Examples of wellness nursing diagnoses have been given. However, these diagnoses represent only a small portion of those that might be developed.

To further the reader's understanding of the use of wellness nursing diagnoses with adolescents, Table 8.1 illustrates the relationships among the diagnoses discussed in this chapter, examples of behaviors appropriate to the diagnoses, and examples of nursing interventions.

References

Erikson, E.H. (1963). *Childhood and Society*, 2nd ed. New York: Norton.

Piaget, J. (1975). *The Construction of Reality in the Child*. New York: Ballentine Books.

Table 8.1. Relationships Among Selected Wellness Nursing Diagnoses, Behaviors, and Interventions: Adolescents

Wellness Nursing Diagnosis	Adolescent Behaviors	Nursing Interventions
Beginning sense of personal identity	Conforms to peer group norms; nonconformity to adult norms	Explain need for personal identity to caregiver
	Finds support in peer group	Help adolescent verbalize personal values
	Tries out new behaviors with peer group	Encourage adolescent to examine personal values compared to those of peer group
Increasing interest in opposite sex	Begins discussing behaviors of members of opposite sex	Explore expectations with adolescent
	Describes expectations of relationships with peers of opposite sex	Suggest to adolescent situations where dating can begin in a safe environment
	Begins dating activities	
Incorporating secondary sex changes into body image	Awareness of sex changes may produce pleasure or displeasure	Let adolescent verbalize feelings about sexual changes

(continued)

139

Wellness Nursing Diagnosis	Adolescent Behaviors	Nursing Interventions
Incorporating secondary sex changes into body image (cont'd.)	Concern over appearance	Encourage caregiver to keep lines of communication open with adolescent
	Experiments with various types of dress, hairstyles, etc.	Correct misconceptions or myths about sexuality and reproduction with adolescent
	Sexual feelings	
Beginning formulation of occupational goals	Describes own strengths and weaknesses, which lead to interest in particular occupations	Explore adolescent's occupational interests
	Seeks resources to learn more about occupations	Provide adolescent with resources about particular occupations
	Begins to describe personal goals	Reinforce development of personal goals with adolescent
Beginning separation from family authority	Peer group dominates interests, time, dress style, and norms for behavior	Explore conflicts between personal and family values with adolescent and/or family
	Questions family values	
	May be argumentative with parents	Reassure adolescent and/or caregiver that this is a normal process
	Confides less in parents	Encourage adolescent to problem solve to

		resolve conflicts
	Expresses need for privacy and autonomy	Explore ways to achieve privacy needs with adolescent and/or caregiver
Increasing consideration of others' opinions	Concerned about others' opinions of them	Listen to adolescent's concerns
	Able to differentiate between own thoughts and those of others	Encourage adolescent to compare own and others' opinions to clarify expectations and increase ability to discriminate between own and others' values
	Able to describe others' opinions accurately	
Increasing ability for abstract reasoning	Ability to logically outline a problem and arrive at a solution	Encourage adolescent to problem solve to resolve conflicts
	Uses facts to defend position	Encourage adolescent to consider consequences of behavior
	Can predict future as well as present events	Reinforce adolescent's decision-making ability
	Can analyze and synthesize material	

(continued)

141

Wellness Nursing Diagnosis	Client Behaviors	Nursing Interventions
Developing potentially long-lasting relationships	Develops one-to-one relationship with same-sex peer	Encourage adolescent to develop relationships to obtain mutual support and encouragement
	Decreases group activities and increases one-to-one activities	
	Tries out new roles and behaviors with one person	
Developing relationships with opposite-sex peers	Explores common interests with opposite-sex peers	Encourage adolescent to discover mutual interests with opposite-sex peers
	Engages in beginning dating in mixed groups	Encourage adolescent to begin dating in order to learn more about self and others of opposite sex as foundation for future relationships
	Participates in double dates or single-pair dates	
	Participates in many phone conversations with opposite-sex peers	

142

| *Increasing personal interests and hobbies* | Particular interests become more important and take up increasingly larger amounts of time | Encourage adolescent to identify and develop personal interests |
| | Interests may direct action toward particular occupation or volunteer activity | Reinforce adolescent's accomplishments in personal interest area |

9
~

Wellness Nursing Diagnoses for Adults: Early Adulthood

Nurses work with adults in a variety of arenas in addition to the acute care setting. Support groups and educative groups are frequently composed of adults of various ages. Occupational health and community health nursing agendas also specify health promotion activities directed toward healthy adults.

As mentioned in Chapter 3, the concept of health promotion includes a variety of activities related to nutritional practices, balance between rest and exercise, use of leisure time, and stress management. The reader is referred to this chapter for general areas of assessment. However, the adult also accomplishes a variety of developmental tasks across the life span that contribute to a sense of well-being. The developmental tasks for the young adult will be discussed in this chapter.

A variety of factors influence attainment of developmental tasks and must be considered during assessment in early adulthood. These factors include age, education, cultural background, and past experiences. Interactions with others, social support, and family patterns for seeking health care or carrying out health promotion activities also influence the adult. Family interaction impacts on how well the individual accomplishes personal developmental tasks. Likewise, expectations of the self, feelings of competence and self-worth, and social expectations play a part in determining the degree to which developmental tasks are attained.

As with previous chapters, the wellness nursing diagnoses presented here represent the first part of the diagnosis (client response). Contributing factors identified in particular client situations will determine the second part of the diagnosis (condition).

~ Assessment of Strengths

In general, early adulthood is defined as 18 to 35 years of age. The task of early adulthood is intimacy (Erikson, 1963). The young adult moves from a major emphasis on developing one's own personal identity, although that is still occurring to some degree, to making attachments to others, resulting in intimate relationships. The ethical strength to make commitments and abide by them is present. During this time, the adult is developing enduring friendships and is seeking a mate, or is married and engaging in the task of beginning a family. The need for human closeness and sexual fulfillment is paramount during this time.

Levinson (1978) considers early adulthood as ages 17 to 45. He states that the person is at the peak of intellectual and physical development at this time. These abilities remain stable until around age 40. During this period, the need to seek personal gratification is high. Over the course of early adulthood, one moves through the novice stage of adulthood, from assuming junior roles at work, beginning marriage and parenting roles, and beginning service to the community, to a more "senior" position at home, work, and in the community.

Milestones that occur during ages 17–45 include entering the adult world (22–28); age 30 transition (changing life structure); settling down (30–40); becoming one's own person (36–40), and midlife transition (40–45). At each of these milestones, the person evaluates his or her life structure and either reaffirms the chosen direction or makes changes in order to achieve the "senior" status mentioned above.

Identity

Combining knowledge gained from both Erikson (1963) and Levinson (1978), it can be seen that the general framework of early adulthood takes a path similar to the one described in the following paragraphs. In the early years of this phase, the adult usually leaves home. Whether going to college, joining the armed services, or joining the work force, the task of separating from the family is taken, with reduction in dependence on family support and authority. Role relationships with parents often change and become more equal. The person engages in warm relationships with peers and family and begins to seek a mate. The person views himself or herself as an adult. Some questions that the nurse might use to assess the young adult related to identity include:

- How does this person interact with parents?
- What kinds of relationships exist with peers?
- Does the client describe himself or herself as an adult?
- Who makes the decisions about the client's personal life?
- Does the client assume responsibility for his or her actions?

Examples of wellness nursing diagnoses pertinent to this time are

~ *Increasing separation from family authority*
~ *Beginning adult identity*

Work and Personal Responsibilities

In addition, the young adult is in the process of selecting an occupation and starting a career. When young adults enter the work world, relationships are developed that might affect their career path. As the adult starts assuming other responsibilities related to home and family, civic and church roles, and leadership in professional organizations, a balance between personal world and work world must be achieved. Assessment questions might include:

- In what kind of community activities does the client participate? Civic organizations? Professional groups? Church?
- How are professional, personal, and family responsibilities balanced?
- What kind of relationships does the client have with co-workers?

Examples of wellness nursing diagnoses would be

- ~ *Assuming leadership role in community*
- ~ *Beginning balance of personal and work responsibilities*
- ~ *Developing relationships within the work force*

Parenting

As this phase continues, the adult often becomes a parent and develops the parenting skills needed for each stage of his or her child's development. Patterns of parenting must be worked out between partners, including rules for discipline as well as division of labor related to the tasks of childrearing such as bathing, feeding, etc. Problem-solving skills are increasingly important as responsibilities increase and new situations are encountered.

Chapter 4 deals with the childbearing family and the wellness diagnoses related to this developmental task. Assessment questions about parenting that might be asked include:

- How has the couple divided parenting tasks?
- How does the client make complex decisions related to parenting and family responsibilities?
- How does the client feel about being a parent?
- How flexible is the client about parenting roles and responsibilities?
- Has the client adjusted parenting activities with the growth of the child?

Wellness nursing diagnoses would include

- ~ *Increasing problem-solving ability*
- ~ *Defining marital role behaviors*
- ~ *Beginning acceptance of parenting role*
- ~ *Reevaluating and developing parenting skills consistent with needs of growing children*

Life-Change Adjustment

Adjustments to life changes have to occur as the adult undertakes career moves, makes career changes, or assumes increased financial responsibilities such as owning a house. Promotions at work may necessitate moving to another location or seeking additional education. The woman who decides to go back to work after her children are in school must balance several roles at one time. As appropriate, the following assessment questions might be asked:

- How has the client adjusted to a career move or a career change?
- Has the client been able to develop relationships with coworkers in the new work setting?
- How has the client adjusted to the need for increased education?
- How does the client balance the demands of work, personal life, and family responsibilities?
- What adjustments have occurred related to increased financial responsibility?
- What kinds of plans does the client have related to long-term security?

Wellness diagnoses would include

~ *Adjusting to career change*
~ *Adjusting to relocation*
~ *Balancing multiple roles*
~ *Developing long-term goals for family security*

CASE STUDY

To illustrate the use of wellness nursing diagnoses in early adulthood, the following case study is presented.

Jeanette is 30 years old, married, and has one child, Bobby, age 4. She works full-time as an accountant. She and her husband have devised a system of child care where they alternate tasks as necessary. She is beginning to anticipate the time that Bobby will go to kindergarten, and realizes that as he grows, his demands for her time and attention will change.

Jeanette works well with her coworkers and is beginning to take some leadership in the organization. In addition, she has begun to sing in her church choir and recently was elected to an office in her professional organization. Although she is tired at times, she states that she is pleased with her professional advancement and thinks that she is a good mother.

Wellness nursing diagnoses for Jeanette include *reevaluating and developing parenting skills consistent with needs of growing children, developing relationships within the work force,* and *beginning balance of personal and work responsibilities.* Goals would include (a) acquisition of new parenting skills as appropriate, (b) continued relationships within the work force, and (c) balance of personal and work responsibilities. Interventions might include provision of information related to growth and development of a 4- and 5-year-old, praise for work-related accomplishments, and discussion of ways to balance multiple roles.

SUMMARY

In summary, a variety of wellness nursing diagnoses, based on the developmental tasks of adults, have been presented for use with the young adult. To provide further information about the relationship of wellness diagnoses to nursing actions, Table 9.1 (see overleaf) illustrates the relationships among the nursing diagnoses presented in this chapter, selected behaviors, and suggested interventions.

References

Erikson, E.H. (1963). *Childhood and Society,* 2nd ed. New York: Norton and Norton.

Levinson, D.J. (1978). *The Seasons of a Man's Life.* New York: Random House.

Table 9.1. Relationships Among Selected Wellness Nursing Diagnoses, Behaviors, and Interventions: Early Adulthood

Wellness Nursing Diagnosis	Early Adulthood Behaviors	Nursing Interventions
Increasing separation from family authority	Seeks parents' opinions regarding choices but assumes responsibility for final behavior	Reinforce independence as appropriate
	Shares experiences with parents and vice versa	Explore alternative actions to aid in decision making
	Makes some decisions without parental input	Encourage communication with family
Beginning adult identity	States he or she is responsible for own actions	Praise independent actions
	Independently manages resources such as time and money	Reinforce decisions as appropriate
	Makes own decisions about housing, lifestyle, etc.	
Assuming leadership role in community	Membership in civic, church, or school organizations	Reinforce interest in community activities
		Explore ways to participate in community

		activities
	Participates in homeowners' organization	Encourage development of leadership skills
	Does volunteer work in community	
	Active in professional organizations	
Beginning balance of personal and work responsibilities	Recognizes need for leisure activities	Reinforce need to balance personal and work activities
	Developing hobbies or other interests outside work-related activities	Help determine interests and provide resources to develop these interests
	Developing personal side of life such as getting married, starting a family, etc.	
Developing relationships within the work force	Developing collegial relationships with coworkers	Reinforce need to network
	Developing plan for career advancement/mobility	Explore career alternatives and ways for advancement
	Begins to assume increasing responsibility at work	Explore options for increased responsibility and ways to gain skills to handle increased responsibility
	Participates in goal development for self and organization as appropriate	

(continued)

Wellness Nursing Diagnosis	Early Adulthood Behaviors	Nursing Interventions
Increasing problem-solving ability	Recognizes need to gain new information or skill	Aid in problem-solving activities by exploring alternatives
	Seeks relevant information to help problem solve in new situations	Aid in clarifying goals
	Considers alternatives to present behavior	Provide information about resources for skill development or goal attainment
	Learns new skills as necessary when new situations arise	
Defining marital role behaviors	Shares views about marriage with mate or prospective mate	Reinforce discussion of views with mate or prospective mate
	Works toward mutually satisfying decisions about roles and division of labor in marriage with mate or prospective mate	Provide information about alternative views or opinions
Beginning acceptance of parenting role	Describes feelings about becoming a new parent	Explore feelings
	Seeks information about parenting behaviors	Explore parenting values and alternatives
	Selects parenting role models and explores	Reinforce information-seeking behaviors

	their views and experiences	Provide information about parenting behaviors or parenting classes
	Shares parenting views with mate and works toward mutually satisfying decisions about parenting roles and activities	
	Prepares for anticipated infant by selecting furniture, clothing, and gathering needed equipment	
Re-evaluating and developing parenting skills consistent with needs of growing children	Recognizes needs of growing children	Praise recognition of differences
	Seeks new parenting skills	Provide information about developmental needs of children
	Alters parenting skills related to child's needs and age	Suggest alternative parenting skills
Adjusting to career change	Describes feelings about career change	Explore feelings about career change
	Recognizes impact of career change on self and/or family	Suggest ways to reduce stress during career change

(continued)

153

Wellness Nursing Diagnosis	Early Adulthood Behaviors	Nursing Interventions
Adjusting to career change (cont'd.)	Begins developing strategies to facilitate adjustment to career change	Suggest strategies to facilitate adjustment to career change or reinforce strategies already being used
Adjusting to relocation	Recognizes impact of relocation on self and/or family	Explore impact of changes on self and/or family
	Reaches out to local resources such as churches, workplace, or schools to learn about new community	Provide information about local resources
		Reinforce reaching-out activities
	Describes positive aspects of relocation	
Balancing multiple roles	Discusses impact of multiple roles on self and/or family	Explore feelings about multiple roles
	Seeks ways to reorganize activities or reduce duplication of effort	Aid in prioritizing activities
		Discuss activities that might be eliminated or assumed by another person
	Seeks help from other family members to accomplish multiple tasks	
	Prioritizes activities and recognizes that some activities may have to be relinquished	

Developing *long-term goals for family security*	Discusses long-term goals with family	Explore realistic goals with client
	Prioritizes goals and makes sure goals are realistic	Aid in prioritization of goals as appropriate
	Creates plan to accomplish goals such as way to buy a house, way to increase savings for college fund, etc.	Discuss strategies for reaching goals

10

~

Wellness Nursing Diagnoses for Adults: Middle Adulthood

Nurses often have contact with clients in middle adulthood in the hospital. Other settings might include wellness centers, support groups, and health education classes.

Chapter 3 presents a general assessment for the adult. However, the adult also accomplishes a variety of developmental tasks across the life span that contribute to a sense of well-being. Chapter 9 describes a variety of factors that influence attainment of developmental tasks in the adult client. The developmental tasks in middle adulthood will be the focus of this chapter.

As with previous chapters, the wellness nursing diagnoses presented here represent the first part of the diagnosis (client response). Contributing factors identified in particular client situations will determine the second part of the diagnosis (condition).

~ Assessment of Strengths

Erikson (1963) states that the period of middle adulthood ranges from approximately 35 to 60 years of age and the developmental task is generativity. Levinson (1978) considers middle adulthood from 45 to 60 and describes this as a time of building new life structures. A midlife transition occurs at 50–55 years of age.

Personal and Family Changes

Major concerns about guiding and developing the next generation emerge in middle adulthood. This time is generally a productive one with much energy placed on career development, family responsibilities for growing children, and community concerns.

Those adults in stable marriages will strengthen family roots while adults in unstable marriages may divorce and remarry, causing lifestyle changes that result in complex family configurations. Other changes in family configurations may occur due to birth, death, children moving out, or moving an aging parent(s) into one's home. Assessment questions related to personal and family changes could include:

- How does the client view his or her own personal growth and accomplishments?
- What kind of community involvement does the client have?
- What events have occurred to foster career development and how has the client adapted to these events?
- What changes have occurred in family size or structure and how has the client adapted to these changes?

Some wellness nursing diagnoses related to this stage include

~ *Pride in accomplishments*
~ *Adapting to the growing family*
~ *Adjusting to changes in family configuration*

Reevaluation Process

This age may also be a time for goal reexamination, accomplishment evaluation, and self-acceptance. As children grow up and leave home, the original couple may have to reestablish their relationship. Women who have been primarily homemakers may have to develop new interests since the "empty nest" may leave them with free time that they do not know how to fill.

Physiological changes that accompany the aging process necessitate adaptation to less energy, annoying memory lapses, or minor aches and pains. Reconsideration of what clients wish to accomplish often occurs as they realize that all their dreams from earlier years have not been fulfilled, nor will it be possible to fulfill them. On the other hand, adults often become more accepting of themselves and no longer feel the necessity of proving themselves to others. With such acceptance comes enjoyment of the chosen lifestyle. Some assessment questions might include:

- What kind of physiological changes has the client experienced?
- What kind of adjustment has been made related to these physiological changes?
- Has the client reevaluated his or her life goals? Is the client satisfied with his or her achievements? How realistic are the goals?

Pertinent wellness diagnoses for these years include

- ~ *Adapting to minor health changes*
- ~ *Reevaluating personal goals*
- ~ *Increasing acceptance of self*

Financial Needs and Aging Parents

Tasks related to financial management emerge when children go to college, health care costs increase, or aging parents can no longer care for themselves. Continued problem solving and stress management related to these areas is necessary. Increasing responsibilities occur as the adults' parents age. In particular, the adult woman "sandwiched" between generations, giving care to both younger and older family members, is clearly affected. Assessment questions related to these issues include:

- What kinds of added financial responsibility is the client experiencing?
- Have plans been made to cover this increased financial responsibility?

- What type of problem solving has been done related to increased financial responsibility?
- What impact do aging parents have on the client and his or her family?
- What is the health status of the client's parents?
- What plans have been made regarding care of the client's aging parents?

Wellness nursing diagnoses might include

~ *Adapting to increased financial responsibilities*
~ *Exploring alternatives for parental care*

Retirement Planning

Toward the end of the middle years, retirement planning emerges. The need for ways to use leisure time, expand outside interests, and redirect life goals occurs. Adjustment to losses may become necessary if parents die. Assessment questions for this area include:

- What changes does the client anticipate about retirement?
- What kind of retirement planning has the client done?
- What interests outside the work environment does the client have that can be pursued upon retirement?

A wellness diagnosis would be

~ *Planning for retirement*

CASE STUDY

To illustrate the use of wellness nursing diagnoses with a client in middle adulthood, the following case study is presented.

Jeremy is a 45-year-old-man who has a wife and three children. One child is in college and a second is a senior in high school. As a construction worker, Jeremy has experienced several minor accidents over the years and now has some arthritis in his knee. He recognizes that he has less energy than he had 10 years ago and remarks that "I don't get as much done as I used to."

Jeremy's mother is a widow who is in fairly good health, but Jeremy observes that her memory is starting to fail and that she is not as active as she used to be. As an only child, he knows that he will be responsible for her care as she ages. He has talked to his mother about this and they have looked at housing for the elderly in his community.

Wellness nursing diagnoses for Jeremy could include *adapting to increased financial responsibilities, adapting to minor health changes,* and *exploring alternatives for parental care.* Goals for Jeremy could include (a) continued adaptation to increased financial responsibilities, (b) continued adaptation to the aging process, and (c) continued planning for parental care. Interventions might include positive reinforcement of ability to manage increased financial responsibilities, exploration of how minor health changes are affecting his lifestyle, and suggestions of possible parental care alternatives.

SUMMARY

In summary, a variety of wellness nursing diagnoses, based on the developmental tasks of the adult, have been presented for use with the adult in middle adulthood. To provide further information about the relationship of wellness diagnoses to nursing actions, Table 10.1 illustrates the relationships among the nursing diagnoses presented in this chapter, selected behaviors, and suggested interventions.

References

Erikson, E.H. (1963). *Childhood and Society,* 2nd ed. New York: Norton and Norton.

Levinson, D.J. (1978). *The Seasons of a Man's Life.* New York: Random House.

Table 10.1. Relationships Among Selected Wellness Nursing Diagnoses, Behaviors, and Interventions: Middle Adulthood

Wellness Nursing Diagnosis	Middle Adulthood Behaviors	Nursing Interventions
Pride in accomplishments	Enumerates accomplishments and expresses satisfaction with them	Praise accomplishments
		Reinforce self-evaluation
	Recognizes and accepts own strengths and weaknesses	Discuss ways to strengthen abilities
	Explores ways to strengthen abilities	
Adapting to the growing family	Reassesses self and/or family needs	Discuss assessment of needs
	Recognizes increased responsibility (additional children, growing children, and the like) and describes impact on self and/or family unit	Discuss needs of growing children
		Help prioritize needs and responsibilities
		Explore ways that needs of family can be met
	Seeks new information and/or skills to meet increased responsibility	Provide information about ways to gain new knowledge or skills

(continued)

161

Wellness Nursing Diagnosis	Middle Adulthood Behaviors	Nursing Interventions
Adapting to the growing family Cont'd.)	Recognizes interaction of family members and impact of change on each one	Praise adjustment
		Reinforce recognition of family interaction
	Considers needs for increased space and privacy	
Adjusting to changes in family configuration	Incorporates new family members into nuclear unit as appropriate	Explore ways to incorporate new family members into household
	Recognizes loss of family members and impact on family unit	Reinforce efforts made to incorporate new family members
		Explore ways to adjust to loss of family members
Adapting to minor health changes	Describes impact of minor health changes on lifestyle	Discuss age-related changes
	Recognizes that changes are inevitable	Reinforce efforts to accommodate
	Accommodates to changes such as making lists to help one's memory, changing exercise routines to increase muscle flexibility, etc.	Explore other alternatives for accommodation

Reevaluating personal goals	Reviews life experiences and goal attainment	Reinforce accomplishments
	Recognizes all dreams may not be accomplished	Assist in reformulation of new or revised goals
	Reassesses present goals and determines reality of meeting them	Explore realistic ways to meet new or revised goals
	Reformulates goals as appropriate	
Increasing acceptance of self	At peace with self; no longer has to live up to expectations of others	Reinforce self-acceptance
	Recognizes all dreams may not be accomplished but expresses satisfaction with level of accomplishment	Reinforce accomplishments
	Recognizes limitations of time and energy level	Suggest reasonable activities given limits of time and energy level
Adapting to increasing financial responsibilities	Evaluates budgetary needs	Discuss increased responsibilities and explore options for meeting those responsibilities

(continued)

163

Wellness Nursing Diagnosis	Middle Adulthood Behaviors	Nursing Interventions
Adapting to increasing financial responsibilities (cont'd.)	Considers options to increase resources or consolidate present resources	
Exploring alternatives for parental care	Recognizes needs of aging parents	Reinforce recognition of needs of both family unit and parents
	Considers needs of family unit as well as needs of aging parents	Provide information on alternative care options
	Evaluates options for care of parents	Facilitate problem solving
Planning for retirement	Evaluates current interests and use of leisure time	Reinforce retirement planning
	Explores new ways to use leisure time	Explore interests and suggest possible alternatives when increased leisure time becomes available
	Develops new hobbies consistent with energy level and physical ability	Reinforce inclusion of family in retirement plans
	Recognizes need to plan for retirement	
	Discusses retirement plans with family	

11

~

Wellness Nursing Diagnoses for Adults: Late Adulthood

Nurses work with older adults in a variety of places in addition to the acute care setting. Day care centers for the elderly have well clients. In addition, support groups and education groups are frequently composed of adults of various ages. A general strength assessment for the adult is described in Chapter 3. Chapter 9 also describes some factors that may influence the adult's ability to complete the developmental tasks for his or her age group. In this chapter, the developmental tasks of the older adult will be discussed.

As with previous chapters, the wellness nursing diagnoses presented here represent the first part of the diagnosis (client response). Contributing factors identified in particular client situations will determine the second part of the diagnosis (condition).

~ Assessment of Strengths

According to both Erikson (1963) and Levinson (1978), late adulthood starts around 60 to 65 years of age and continues until the end of life. The developmental task of late adulthood is ego integrity (Erikson, 1963). Part of this task is accepting what one has done as worthwhile regardless of the pain and struggles incurred along the way. Many adjustments may arise resulting from retirement, death of loved ones, declining health, and less income.

Retirement

The early part of this stage focuses on retirement and how to use leisure time. If the adult's identity has come primarily from the work role, a search for new ways to feel valued and worthwhile may be needed. Learning new skills, developing new interests, or reviving old interests may be ways to feel a sense of accomplishment. Family relationships, particularly spousal, may have to be redefined since the couple has more time together. Some assessment questions that the nurse might ask include:

- What kinds of adjustment has the client or family made related to retirement?
- How does the client feel about himself or herself since retirement?
- Does the client enjoy retirement?
- What goals does the client have?
- In what kinds of leisure activities does the client participate?
- What kind of relationship does the client has with his or her spouse?
- What kinds of activities do the couple participate in together?

Wellness diagnoses include

~ *Adapting to retirement*
~ *Reestablishing spousal relationships*

Health Care Concerns

Concern with health care increases during this stage. As health and strength decline, adjustments must be made. Adaptation to chronic illness may also be necessary. When examining health-promoting lifestyles, Walker, Volkan, Sechrist, and Pender (1988) found that older adults (aged 55–88) scored significantly higher on the dimension of health responsibility than middle-aged and young adults. Health responsibility was defined as "attending to and accepting responsibility for one's health, being educated about health, and seeking professional assistance as necessary" (p. 80). When older adults seek information about how to deal with changes in health status, they incorporate this information into their lifestyles and continue as many of the same activities as possible. Assessment questions might include:

- What changes in health status is the client experiencing?
- What effect have these changes had on lifestyle?
- How does the client assume responsibility for his or her own health care?
- What sources of information does the client use to assess his or her health? To seek health care?

Wellness nursing diagnoses for this age group would be

~ *Progressive adjustment to physiological changes*
~ *Assuming responsibility for own health*

Resiliency and Flexibility

Although changes become more frequent as a person ages, the active older adult, 75+, adjusts to these changes by recognizing that life is transitory at best. Limited energy restricts the older adult who then must be selective about how that energy is spent. Long-term plans diminish and enjoyment is gained from day-to-day living.

Although new friends cannot replace the old, pleasure can be achieved from new relationships. Because wisdom has developed from going through difficult times, the older adult has the flexibility and resiliency needed to find joy in the immediate situation.

Although the outsider might view the older adult's life as fairly restrictive, most older adults describe themselves as active and healthy despite chronic illness or physical disabilities. People with a terminal diagnosis are able to look at the positive aspects of their life and describe themselves as healthy as long as they can do the things they desire (Fryback, 1993).

In a study of older adults, Ruffing-Rahal (1989) found three core themes of well-being: activity, affirmation, and synthesis. They choose meaningful activities that often involve challenges or personal development as they learn new skills. Older adults often spend time in service to others, which provides social involvement as well as meaning to their lives. Lastly, older adults develop some sort of meaningful pattern to their daily lives. No longer having work schedules to organize their time, they find other ways to incorporate a routine into daily living. Self-care activities often are part of this pattern, especially if they maintain autonomy. Assessment questions related to client flexibility and resiliency include:

- How does the client set priorities for an activity?
- Does the client have an established pattern of daily living?
- How flexible is the client with regard to this pattern?
- What gives the client enjoyment?
- How does the client view his or her health state?
- In what community activities is the client engaged?

Wellness nursing diagnoses that would apply to these older adults include

~ *Participating in satisfying activities*
~ *Developing a pattern for daily living*
~ *Involvement in service activities*

The second theme, affirmation, deals with the older adult's evaluation of his or her own life. In general, Ruffing-Rahal (1989) found that older adults thought their life had meaning and they were able to meet some of their personal goals. They also remained optimistic about their present life, stating that they were thankful to be alive and were hopeful about each new day. Assessment questions related to affirmation include:

- Does the client think his or her life has meaning?
- What kinds of activity does the client say give meaning to life?
- What gives the client hope?

- Is the client able to meet personal goals? If so, in what way?

A wellness nursing diagnosis related to these feelings might be

~ *Satisfaction with past and present life as lived*

Ruffing-Rahal's (1989) third theme, synthesis, reflects a blending of life experiences into a pattern of resiliency where adults realize they have lived through good and bad times and have survived both. Subjects recounted that they had "learned to live a day at a time and to accept things as they are" (p. 16). Assessment questions related to resiliency might include:

- What is the client's philosophy about life?
- What personal strengths can the client describe?
- Does the client deal with one day at a time?

A wellness diagnosis related to this theme would be

~ *Increasing recognition of one's own strengths.*

CASE STUDY

To illustrate the use of wellness nursing diagnoses with an older adult, the following case study is presented.

J.B. is an 81-year-old man with a medical diagnosis of stage IV Hodgkin's lymphoma for which he is currently undergoing chemotherapy.

J.B. lives in his own home with his wife of 62 years, enjoys fishing, maintains a vegetable garden, and has an active social life. The couple have one married son, two grandchildren, and three great-grandchildren.

J.B. has an active sense of humor manifested by telling jokes to the nurse visiting his home. He openly expresses affection to his wife. He takes pride in his past accomplishments, stating, "I have always worked hard and made my own way." Because of good financial management, he has good health care coverage and no money worries.

J.B. is very optimistic about his prognosis and believes he has several more years to live. He does express some concern about his wife if anything should happen to him. Currently, he has had a 30-pound weight loss and has experienced some fatigue. A review of systems reveals good physical health except for the lymphoma.

J.B. states his goal is to "regain my strength, gain some weight, and be able to continue gardening and fishing." He actively seeks information about ways to gain weight and foods to eat that will provide optimum nutrition. He asks questions about his chemotherapy such as, "What will the drugs to do me?" and discusses his wishes to know the outcomes of the chemotherapy.

Even though he has cancer, the overall picture of J.B.'s situation is a positive one. He still carries out an independent role as provider, father, and mate; maintains family and social relationships; and participates in hobbies such as gardening and fishing. Several wellness nursing diagnoses that would be appropriate for this client are *assuming responsibility for own health, participating in satisfying activities,* and *continued satisfaction with past and present life as lived.*

Client-centered goals for J.B. would be (a) increased knowledge about ways to meet health care needs and (b) continued participation in satisfying activities. Nursing interventions would include provision of information about health status, medical regimen, and ways to maintain his current state of health and/or improve it as much as possible. Information would be presented at the pace that is comfortable for the client and would include consideration of the client's wishes, environment, and lifestyle in order to find realistic ways for the client to continue to be independent and responsible for his own health. Exploration of activities that the client finds satisfying and is able to carry out, or identification of new activities if past activities are no longer possible, would facilitate achievement of the second goal.

SUMMARY

In summary, a variety of wellness nursing diagnoses, based on the developmental tasks of the adult, have been presented for use with the adult in late adulthood. To provide further information about the relationship of wellness diagnoses to nursing actions, Table 11.1 (see overleaf) illustrates the relationships among the nursing diagnoses presented in this chapter, selected behaviors, and suggested interventions.

References

Erikson, E.H. (1963). *Childhood and Society*, 2nd ed. New York: Norton and Norton.

Fryback, P.B. (1993). Health for people with a terminal diagnosis. *Nursing Science Quarterly*, 6(3), 147–159.

Levinson, D.J. (1978). *The Seasons of a Man's Life*. New York: Random House.

Ruffing-Rahal, M.A. (1989). Ecological well-being: A study of community-dwelling older adults. *Health Values*, 13(1), 10–19.

Walker, S.N., Volkan, K, Sechrist, K.R., and Pender, N.J. (1988). Health-promoting life styles of older adults: Comparisons with young and middle-aged adults, correlates and patterns. *Advances in Nursing Science*, 11(1), 76–90.

Table 11.1. Relationships Among Selected Wellness Nursing Diagnoses, Behaviors, and Interventions: Late Adulthood

Wellness Nursing Diagnosis	Late Adulthood Behaviors	Nursing Interventions
Adapting to retirement	Plans use of leisure time, which encourages self-fulfillment	Encourage self-fulfilling activities
	Seeks new and challenging interests or revives old interests	Explore ways to develop new or revived interests
	May seek second career depending on age at retirement	Provide information about community activities for senior adults
Reestablishing spousal relationship	Recognizes need to incorporate spouse into retirement plans	Reinforce recognition of spouse's needs as well as one's own
	Spends time with spouse pursuing mutual interests	Explore activities that would be mutually satisfying for couple
Progressive adjustment to physiological changes	Recognizes physical limitations	Provide information about age-related changes
	Makes environmental changes to accommodate physical changes	Differentiate between normal changes and life-threatening ones
	Recognizes signs and symptoms of declining	

	health and seeks professional help as needed	Suggest accommodations that maximize ability and adaptation
	Maintains appropriate level of independence	Provide list of resources that can provide help as needed
	Seeks information about chronic illness to facilitate adaptation	
Assuming responsibility for own health	Seeks information about health promotion and/or disease condition	Reinforce health-seeking behaviors
	Seeks medical care as appropriate	Provide information as needed
	Engages in health promotion activities	Provide information about referrals for health care as needed
	Incorporates knowledge about illness into lifestyle	Clarify misunderstandings or misconceptions
		Explore ways knowledge can be used to make adaptations to chronic or acute illness
Participating in satisfying activities	Participates in social activities with family and friends	Reinforce outside interests
		Explore realistic alternatives within physical limitations

(continued)

173

Wellness Nursing Diagnosis	Late Adulthood Behaviors	Nursing Interventions
Participating in satisfying activities (cont'd.)	Continues hobbies or other interests within physical limitations	Encourage reminiscence
	Finds joy in short-term activities without long-term planning	Listen to life review
	Expresses satisfaction with life despite limitations	
	At peace with self and God	
	Uses time to the fullest within parameters of health restrictions	
	Reminisces about life events	
Developing a pattern for daily living	Recognizes need to have a plan for the day in order to maintain meaning for life as well as social interaction	Explore what activities are meaningful
		Help select activities within level of functioning and energy level
	Plans daily activities	
	Establishes a routine for activities of daily living such as exercise, etc.	Reinforce maintaining a daily routine

Involvement in service activities	States need to be involved in doing for others	Reinforce interest in helping others
	Selects several activities that would be meaningful to fulfill this need	Provide information about volunteer/community options
	Participates in activities that help meet needs of others, i.e., church, service organizations, etc.	Explore realistic goals for service activities
Satisfaction with past and present life as lived	Verbalizes satisfaction with past life and experiences	Review satisfying experiences
	Expresses optimism about approaching each day	Reinforce participation in satisfying activities
	Finds satisfaction in current activities	Help identify positive aspects of life
Increasing recognition of one's own strengths	Identifies areas of past and present strengths	Reinforce client strengths
	Modifies activities to use present strengths to the fullest	Discuss ways to modify living patterns to use present strengths

(continued)

175

Wellness Nursing Diagnosis	Late Adulthood Behaviors	Nursing Interventions
Increasing recognition of one's own strengths (cont'd.)	Lives one day at a time and maintains control over areas of life where control is possible	Explore areas that client can still control
		Encourage letting go of those areas that client cannot control
		Reinforce living for the day rather than worrying about limitations in the future

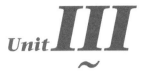

Unit **III**
~

Wellness Nursing Diagnosis in Special/Selected Health Care Environments

~

12

~

Wellness Nursing Diagnoses for Adults in Critical Care

C lients who are acutely ill and admitted to a critical care unit have pathophysiologic disruptions to one or more major organ systems. Assessments of these clients are likely to conclude with a list of problem-oriented diagnoses that mirror these pathophysiological states. Besides the physical realm, psychological difficulties and behavioral problems may occur as the client attempts to cope with the physiological and environmental stressors. Current critical care texts and journal articles emphasize the problem-oriented approach. While authors may point out individual patient strengths that facilitate recovery, few identify wellness-oriented diagnoses. In this chapter, we will discuss positive attributes of acutely ill clients and suggest ways to refocus on client strengths and wellness diagnoses. Although other chapters in this book have only included the first portion of the wellness diagnosis (response), we have included the second portion (condition) as well for some diagnoses. Conditions, however, may vary depending on individual client situations.

~ Assessment of Strengths

Health–illness may be viewed as a phenomenon existing on parallel continua along several dimensions: biological, psychological, sociological, spiritual. A client may be far out on the illness end of the biological continuum, yet with adequate sociological resources may express high-level wellness on the psychological and spiritual dimensions. Thus, even when severely ill, many clients demonstrate behavior that can be viewed as a strength and that supports wellness diagnoses. The latter behaviors typically reflect motivation, skill, and knowledge: attributes used by the client to initiate or participate in interventions that will alleviate the pathophysiological or psychological problem or maintain a steady state.

~ Four Areas of Assessment for Wellness Diagnosis

Roberts (1986) proposes a framework for assessment and nursing diagnoses in the critically ill adult composed of four areas: behavior, emotion, environment, and physiology (BEEP). Although the framework was written with a problem-oriented focus, it provides a comprehensive frame of reference for discovery and discussion of wellness-oriented diagnoses. The model remains representative of critical-care nursing practice and is consistent with the systems models of other nursing theorists such as Roy and Andrews (1991) and Neuman (1989), as well as contemporary authors of critical care texts such as Dossey, Guzzetta, and Kenner (1992). An in-depth assessment and comprehensive list of diagnoses in each of these dimensions is beyond the scope of this chapter. However, examples will reflect phenomena commonly found among clients in intensive care units and will provide principles the reader can use to identify additional diagnoses.

Behavior

The behavior components include consciousness, consistency of behavior, characteristics of the client's background, and control of movement.

Consciousness This behavior component includes thought processes and communication. Nurses assess level of consciousness and orientation for signs of deteriorating circulatory or neurological condition or metabolic derangement. Clients who exhibit wellness behaviors in this area are alert, oriented, cooperative, and are able to concentrate, remember, and make reasonable decisions about their care. Clients may recognize episodic confusion related to pain medications, and collaborate with the nurse to establish dosages and schedules of medication adequate to manage pain, yet not impair consciousness. Clients who require *prn* oxygen may request that the oxygen cannula be placed within reach for use during activities that elicit shortness of breath. Clients who are at risk for disorientation related to sensory overload may take action to maintain orientation by seeking out the meaning of sounds and events in the environment or by making specific requests for periods of undisturbed sleep. In these situations, nurses support client decisions and follow through with client requests for specific assistance. Key questions for assessment may include:

- What is the client's score on the mental status exam? On the Glasgow coma scale?
- What client behaviors indicate ability to manage symptoms and prevent altered levels of consciousness?

A state of consciousness and the ability to function cognitively reflect normal aspects of physiological status. These strengths enable the client to communicate and participate in care. Therefore, a wellness diagnosis reflecting these strengths would be

~ *Maintaining consciousness and cognitive function*

The ability to communicate effectively despite impediments such as dyspnea, endotracheal intubation, neurological impairment, or trauma is a major strength and provides an important buffer against anxiety, frustration, and maladaptive coping behaviors. Clients who are dyspneic or who are intubated can communicate through alternate methods such as writing notes or using a letter board. Laryngectomy clients may use electronic speaking devices. Clients with sensory impairments request their glasses and hearing aids in order to facilitate communication. The ability to maintain effective communication also may augment adaptive coping mechanisms by providing a means to channel frustration and anxiety. Nurses support these behaviors by assisting clients to identify and use alternative communication methods and by ensuring that sensory aids and communication tools are within reach and in working order. Important assessment parameters are:

- What methods of communication does the client use? To what extent are these methods effective?
- To what extent are verbal and nonverbal messages congruent?
- To what extent does the client possess sufficient attention span, memory, and strength to use adapted modes of communication (e.g., letter boards, pencil and paper, pantomime)?
- To what extent does the client need and use aids such as eyeglasses and hearing aids?

Clients with strengths in this area manifest congruent verbal and nonverbal communication. They maintain relevant, meaningful interactions with family and caregivers. A wellness diagnosis for this area would be

~ *Maintaining effective communication*

Consistency of Behavior   Consistency of behavior includes compliance and the degree to which the client's behavior is nonviolent and predictable. Sudden changes in behavior, or behavior inconsistent or inappropriate to the situation, may reflect neurologic or metabolic abnormalities, or psychological states such as anxiety, anger, or depression. From a physiologic standpoint, behavior consistency is a strength, depicting a normal neurological or metabolic state. Clients who demonstrate consistency of behavior are those who react in the expected fashion to stimuli in the environment, are cooperative, and do not pose a threat to themselves or others. However, behaviors representing emotional distress may also be viewed as a strength, if appropriate to the situation or if representing the expected developmental process. For example, expression of anger about loss of lower extremity function is an expected reaction for the client with a spinal cord injury and indicates movement in the process from shock and disbelief to working through and acceptance. The nurse supports this stage, providing a safe environment to ventilate feelings and voice concerns.

Although moderate anxiety to panic generally represents a problem, mild anxiety may stimulate motivation for a preventive or therapeutic action—a strength. For example, mild anxiety may provide the motivation necessary for a client with an acute exacerbation of pulmonary disease who is malnourished to drink supplemental high-protein formula in order to increase pulmonary muscle strength. This positive action may improve oxygenation and prevent the need for endotracheal intubation and/or feeding tube placement. The nurse assists the client to remain motivated by helping the client set realistic goals, by providing positive reinforcement for the client's efforts, and by providing necessary equipment and supplies. Questions asked by the nurse to assess consistency of behavior might include:

- To what extent is the client's behavior consistent from day to day?
- To what extent does the client's behavior reflect expected developmental tasks or stages?

Wellness nursing diagnoses for the above situations would be

~ *Progressing through the grieving process*
~ *Maintaining muscle strength related to high motivation to meet nutritional needs*

Persons who believe they are susceptible to the illness, believe that the therapies prescribed will ameliorate or improve the illness state, and perceive they are capable of carrying out the therapies are more likely to participate in the prescribed plan. Provided the treatment plan is appropriate for the medical problem, clients who actively participate in the prescribed activity, fluid restrictions, etc., are also actively and positively progressing toward a wellness state. Assessment questions include:

- To what extent does the client ask about and participate in the prescribed plan of care?
- What is the client's perception of his or her illness process and potential effectiveness of the plan of care?

For those clients who participate in the prescribed plan of care and follow their treatment plan, a wellness diagnosis could be

~ *Complying with the treatment plan*

Characteristics of Client Background Personal idiosyncrasies including diversional activities, knowledge, family process, role function, and sexual function are included in this behavior component. There are certain groups of clients, such as those in the ICU awaiting organ transplant or those recovering from a long illness, who are at risk for boredom and apathy. The nurse assists clients to explore possible diversional activities and acquires items to support these activities. Assessment questions might include

- What kinds of interests or hobbies does the client have?
- How does the client usually spend free time?
- What methods has the client used in the past to alleviate anxiety or boredom?

For those clients who are able to allay anxiety, reduce boredom, and avoid apathy, a wellness diagnosis could be

~ *Facilitating own emotional balance related to initiation of diversional activities*

Many clients "monitor" the environment by asking many questions about the plan of care, various interventions, and procedures. In fact, they often ask the same questions of different caregivers. For clients with this coping style, knowledge about their condition and plan of care allows them to maintain some control over the situation, channel energy, and reduce anxiety. Nurses support this coping mechanism by answering questions patiently and consistently, in the depth and scope appropriate to the client's level of education and curiosity. Questions that nurses might ask of themselves or their clients include:

- What kinds of questions is this client asking?
- Is there a pattern found among the questions asked?
- Who has the client approached with questions?
- How does the client respond when given an answer? Does an answer reduce anxiety?
- How does the client use the information?

Clients who use knowledge as a coping mechanism could have the following wellness nursing diagnosis:

~ *Acquiring knowledge*

Approaching the critical care client from a perspective that includes strengths as well as problems allows nurses to view client care outcomes differently. For example, the nurse may view a client's persistent questioning of each aspect of his or her care as a positive coping strategy for stressful situations. Using a positive approach rather than a problem approach (potential anxiety related to fear of the unknown) acknowledges the client's active participation in managing the situation. Nursing interventions may be designed to support client participation by incorporating explanations and teaching into each new aspect of care as often as necessary. For this client a wellness nursing diagnosis might be

~ *Questioning care related to personal coping style*

Control of Movement   Both tolerance of activity levels and physical mobility (actions associated with an intact neurological and musculoskeletal function) are included in this behavior component. Clients who are motivated to gradually increase time sitting up in a chair, ambulation distance, number of strengthening exercises, etc., exhibit strengths. These self-initiated efforts often are difficult for the client, who may have to overcome pain, fatigue, and dyspnea. The nurse supports the client to sustain these efforts through close monitoring (safety), provision of appropriate support appliances, frequent encouragement, and positive feedback. Assessment questions might include:

- How motivated is the client to increase activity?
- What ways does the client use to sustain increased activity efforts without creating other problems?
- What progressive efforts is the client making regarding mobility and activity tolerance?

These clients would have the following wellness nursing diagnosis:

~ *Improving activity tolerance*

Emotions

The second area of Robert's (1986) BEEP model is the emotional element. This area includes components such as depersonalization, the frustration of helplessness, and despair.

Certainly, it is common in critical care for clients to express feelings of loss of control and powerlessness. Roberts (1986) also identifies feelings of loneliness, frustration, anger, depression, fear of loss, alteration in self-concept, separation, failure to accept, and failure to be personalized.

In Chapter 3, Dr. Stolte suggests that to have strengths, one must first be motivated. This assumption also is true for the critically ill client. In order for the client to effectively relieve feelings of powerlessness, he or she must be motivated to take control when it is offered. Wellness-oriented behaviors indicating attempts to maintain control include frequent requests for information about the illness process and alternative therapies, direct confrontation with staff and physicians, and requests to negotiate routines and therapies. Even the ventilator-dependent client can resume some control over activities of daily living if motivated and given the opportunity. Nurses can increase decision control and decrease feelings of powerlessness by allowing the client to express concerns, fears, and anxieties, by encouraging the client to set goals, and by allowing the client to make as many decisions as possible. Assessment questions to address may include:

- In what situations does the client feel powerless?
- What environmental and staff characteristics inadvertently reinforce feelings of powerlessness?
- What client actions and behaviors depict attempts to remain in control?

For clients who exhibit behaviors that allow them to regain or maintain control, the following wellness diagnosis might be useful:

~ *Retaining sense of control related to ability (opportunity) to make decisions concerning health care*

Feelings of loneliness and separation are typical. Clients are isolated within the confines of a busy, noisy, foreign environment, stripped of their belongings, and cut off from family and friends by restrictive visiting policies. Clients who are successful at overcoming loneliness find alternative activities, such as watching television, reading a Bible, and visiting with housekeepers and staff. They may request extra visiting time for their closest relatives (e.g., spouse, children), communicate with family by telephone, and/or request that family photos or pictures drawn by children/grandchildren be displayed on the wall. Strengths include strong relationships with close family members, with the client receiving support and encouragement during hospitalization. Nurses support clients' efforts through liberal visiting policies, maintaining familiar routines, placing personal belongings in view, and reframing the illness experience as a temporary situation with growth opportunities. Assessment parameters include:

- Has the client experienced loneliness previously and how was the experience resolved?
- To what extent do family and friends visit during visiting hours? How strong is the client–family relationship?
- What are the client's reactions during visitation and when alone? What activities does the client use to pass the time when alone?

Associated wellness diagnoses are

~ *Maintaining social support networks*
~ *Maintaining family cohesiveness*

Self-concept is often disrupted in the critically ill client. Loss of function, loss of bodily part, or disfigurement may add to the stress of a severe physiological problem. However, self-concept may also remain intact, even in the event of serious illness. Clients who maintain a positive self-concept may be those whose basic values and primary motivators are not dependent on body image or physical function. Clients are more likely to maintain a positive self-concept when they perceive the immediate illness and/or role changes to be temporary. However, some clients who must incorporate the chronic illness trajectory or role changes into their future are able to identify positive features of self and maintain a positive self-concept. The nurse assists this process by reinforcing positive attributes and supporting the client's attempts to reframe the illness trajectory. Assessment parameters may include:

- What comments does the client make about his or her illness and its possible consequences for the future?
- To what extent is the client willing/able to discuss the illness? Able to focus on the topic? Willing to make eye contact?
- To what extent does the client participate in self-care?
- To what extent does the client eat meals? Participate in therapies?

A wellness nursing diagnosis related to this area would be

~ *Maintaining consistent self-concept related to realistic, objective appraisal of event*

Acceptance of the medical diagnosis (illness label) and the consequences of the illness is a strength, as it allows the client to move forward and begin to incorporate potential role and lifestyle changes. Psychological energy can be channeled into efforts toward recovery, new learning, and adaptation. Assessment questions related to acceptance of limitations include:

- What kind of statements does the client make about his or her illness?
- How is the client incorporating knowledge about the illness into conversation with family members and others?
- Has the client described any illness-related lifestyle changes that may be necessary?

A wellness diagnosis could be

~ *Accepting limitations from illness/injury*

Environment

Roberts (1986) addresses the environmental component as having the potential to channel the client's progress toward an affirmative or destructive outcome. This section includes sensory overload, sensory deprivation, sleep deprivation, and stress. Granted, machinery noise, small, cramped quarters, and frequent interruption are often not avoidable. However, through coordination of care, environmental stimuli may be diminished. Clients may be able to control their environment by negotiating quiet/rest periods with staff or by requesting that their physicians write orders to omit routine vital signs and procedures during the night. Clients who are able to ask questions about the environment and receive feedback regarding their interpretation of sounds and events may have less potential for confusion. Those who feel more secure in the environment are less likely to suffer anxiety. Normal cognitive function and low anxiety states are strengths that facilitate the healing process. Assessment pertinent to this area includes:

- To what extent does the client interpret sounds and events in the unit correctly? Keep track of time?
- How many hours is the client sleeping per day? REM sleep?
- What is the client's mood state?

Wellness-oriented diagnoses reflecting strengths in this area might be

> ~ *Maintaining sensory input balance*
> ~ *Obtaining normal sensory input*
> ~ *Maintaining usual sleep/rest cycle*

Physiology

In the BEEP model, physiological components include sclera color and status of pupils, skin color, status of central venous pressure, systolic and diastolic blood pressure, chest, lung, and bowel sounds, and status (rate, rhythm, and regularity) of major systems: cardiovascular, pulmonary, renal, neurological, endocrine, and gastrointestinal. Standard assessment protocols are designed to identify actual or potential problems in these physiologic areas. In general, the absence of abnormal findings reflects a strength for that particular system. However, there are some circumstances in which abnormal signs and symptoms are found, yet regulation of pathophysiologic states is occurring, preventing further problems or actively restoring normal function.

For example, a group of clients may be recovering uneventfully due to preventive or restorative practices in which they actively engage. For clients recovering from a myocardial infarction, the myocardium is damaged and is undergoing repair (an abnormality); however, by limiting activity to a certain prescribed level and managing anxiety, the client decreases heart work (energy needs for activity and sympathetic nervous system function). Clients who follow this treatment plan and take responsibility for their own activities are exhibiting strengths. An example of a wellness diagnosis for these clients is

~ *Progressive healing of myocardium related to reduction of physical activity and management of stress response (Stolte, 1989)*

For many clients, multiple medications prescribed to treat pathological conditions result in another set of symptoms. Clients may successfully overcome one such problem, orthostatic hypotension, by such sympathetic nervous system manipulation actions as changing position slowly and engaging in range-of-motion (ROM) exercises. The ability to make changes in one physiological area, which positively affects another area, is a client strength. A related wellness diagnosis would be

~ *Maintaining normal blood pressure during position changes*

Client participation in preventive practices also reflects client strengths. For nurses who have identified problem areas, yet want to focus on positive aspects of patient behavior, recognition of these strengths can accomplish that goal. Wellness diagnoses can reflect client participation in therapy and willingness to be a partner in health care. Examples of such diagnoses are

~ *Effective airway clearance related to independent use of incentive spirometer*
~ *Maintaining skin integrity related to active range of motion and position changes*

These wellness diagnoses are much more client oriented than, for example, "potential for airway occlusion related to stasis of secretions."

Clients may continue to demonstrate a physiologic problem, such as inadequate oxygenation, yet have an associated identified strength. For instance, a client on a ventilator can make efforts that will facilitate the weaning process. For those clients, a wellness diagnosis might be

~ *Progressive weaning from ventilator related to active effort to slow breathing and manage anxiety (Stolte, 1989)*

Although the client may be malnourished, he or she may be actively engaged in correcting the negative state. A wellness diagnosis reflecting this situation might be

~ *Progressing toward nutritional balance related to consistent intake of "x" number of calories/day*

In addition, some clients may exhibit signs and symptoms that signify pathology, yet are able to maintain function at a level that is optimum for them. This situation may warrant wellness diagnoses such as

~ *Sustained ability to carry out self-care activities related to use of pursed-lip breathing (or energy conservation techniques)*
~ *Progressing toward fluid and electrolyte balance related to regulation of fluid intake*

CASE STUDY

Mr. Adams is a 58-year-old white male admitted to the coronary care unit 10 weeks ago with the medical diagnosis of cardiomyopathy. His previous medical history included an anterior wall myocardial infarction with subsequent three-vessel coronary artery bypass grafting (CABG). Postsurgery, he developed gastrointestinal bleeding and required a partial gastrectomy. The abdominal incision became infected with *Candida albicans* and was left open for packing and healing by secondary intention. When discharged from the hospital to his wife's care, he had an open abdominal wound, had lost 60 pounds, required a wheelchair for mobility, and had limited ROM due to prolonged bed rest and immobility. As he relates this history, he states, "They sent me home to die, but here I am, 8 years later!" He and his wife describe his successful convalescence, which included upper and lower body exercises, wound care, and nutritional interventions. One intervention used by Mrs. Adams and her son was to paint a line on the driveway, indicating every gain made in ambulation distance. He describes pushing himself to do the exercises, even though each new set of exercises and increase in repetitions left his muscles sore. Neither Mr. nor Mrs. Adams were boastful in their presentation of the story, yet seemed to take pride in their ability to overcome such obstacles.

Currently, Mr. Adams is awaiting cardiac transplant. His hemodynamic status is maintained with intravenous nitroglycerin, dopamine, and heparin. He also receives several oral medications and an inhalant. He knows the actions, side effects, and times for all of his medications. He takes his medidose inhaler and nose drops independently. He wears humidified oxygen per nasal cannula at 2 L/min. Systolic blood pressure is maintained at 95–105 mmHg. Heart rate averages 75–80 with regular rhythm. There are no gallops, murmurs, or rubs. Respiratory rate is 20 and regular without effort. Lungs are clear to auscultation. He has no chest pain or shortness of breath at an activity level of 2–3 metabolic equivalents (METs). He wears socks to keep his feet warm. Pedal pulses are present and +2. There are old well-healed scars along the inner aspect of both lower legs from removal of superficial veins for his CABG. Hair distribution along lower legs is present but sparse. There is no leg or ankle edema. As he describes the situation, "I feel pretty good now as compared to when I first came in, but if you took away all these (intravenous) medicines, I would go downhill fast."

He is able to get to the chair and toilet in his room independently, feed himself, brush his teeth, and shave, and requires minimal assistance with bathing (2–3 METs). He rests between activities. Mrs. Adams visits daily and the two have developed a bathing and personal hygiene routine, in which she allows him to do whatever activity he can, and assists only as necessary.

Mr. Adams recently had a PIC line inserted to facilitate giving the IV medications and for blood drawing. This "line" is a long IV catheter threaded via the antecubital vein into a central vein that can be left in place for up to 6 months. He is quite "thankful for the line" as he was having new IVs inserted almost every day due to infiltration or phlebitis. The PIC lines are new to the agency, and many of the nurses are unfamiliar with them. Mr. Adams has an excellent understanding of the catheter placement, uses, and maintenance protocols. He is quick to inform any nurse new to his care that he will talk him or her through the procedure for drawing blood, etc., through the line. He was quite assertive about insisting that nurses draw blood through the line rather than "stick" him for a blood sample, and could give the rationale for all blood samples including coagulation studies. To ensure that all nurses use the PIC line for obtaining blood samples, he asked the physician to "write an order" on the chart.

Because Mr. Adams and his wife complete much of his personal care, and his physical status is "stable" on the current regimen, nursing tasks are minimal: 4-hour assessments, vital signs, and medication administration. His private room is across from the nurse's station, and he often smiles and waves at the nurses as they pass by. The nurses have a positive regard for Mr. Adams and his wife and drop by to visit for a few minutes throughout the day. Mr. Adams is quiet and doesn't call for the nurses often, but enjoys visiting with them as they drop in.

Mr. and Mrs. Adams have met two other heart transplant patients and their spouses (one is doing well, the other has suffered a series of complications). They have kept in contact with the other families and have followed the ups and downs of the posttransplant trajectory vicariously. Mr. Adams states, "I'll have been in here 10 weeks tomorrow." It gets "a little old, being in the unit, but it's not too bad." If he wakes up at night and is feeling a little depressed he just "gets up and turns on the light and reads or does some activity." If the TV program he is watching is depressing, he "just changes the channel." After all, he states, "It's not over until you give up." He explained that he was now in "category one" and "number one" on the waiting list for a heart. In fact, there had been a heart available several weeks ago, "but my surgeon turned it down because it wasn't quite good enough for me. He (Dr. P.) wanted a little stronger heart." This concern by the surgeon for the best possible heart seemed to be reassuring to Mr. Adams.

Although Mr. Adams is critically ill, requiring hospitalization and intravenous pharmacologic support to maintain cardiac function, he exhibits many strengths and is actively involved in his care. In the physiologic realm he demonstrates *independence in (most) self-care activities related to use of energy conservation principles.* Nursing interventions include positive reinforcement for use of energy conservation techniques, and organization of nursing care to fit within the client's capabilities and time sequences.

In the psychological realm Mr. Adams demonstrates *decision control in care related to knowledge about pathological state and treatment plans* and *adaptive coping with imposed physical and environmental restrictions related to hope.* For the first diagnosis, the nurse recognizes that the client actively seeks information in order to participate in care decisions, and thus offers explanations and written or verbal information about all new medications, treatments, etc., recommended or prescribed. The nurse also positively reinforces the knowledge-seeking attribute. Interventions to maintain hope include emphasizing the clients' strengths, recalling previous instances in which the client overcame obstacles, allowing the client to discuss aspects of the current situation that are hopeful and hopeless, and assisting the client to focus on the hopeful aspect. The nurse also supports family relationships by allowing extended family visits.

SUMMARY

Although patients admitted to critical care units are likely to present more problems than strengths, focus on the strengths and assistance with wellness behaviors is an important aspect of holistic nursing care. In this chapter, possible wellness nursing diagnoses relevant to behavior, emotion, environment, and physiology domains are suggested. Associated behaviors and suggested interventions for these diagnoses are presented in Table 12.1. Although wellness diagnoses have been illustrated using two-part format (human response related to factors maintaining the human response), we have chosen to present only the human response portion of the diagnoses in Table 12.1

REFERENCES

Dossey, B.M., Guzzetta, C.E., and Kenner, C.V. (1992). *Critical Care Nursing, Body—Mind—Spirit*, 3rd ed. New York: Lippincott.

Neuman, B. (1989). *The Neuman Systems Model*, 2nd ed. East Norwalk, CT: Appleton-Century-Crofts.

Roberts, S. (1986). *Behavioral Concepts and the Critically Ill Patient*, 2nd ed. Norwalk, CT: Appleton-Century-Crofts.

Roberts, S. (1987). *Nursing Diagnosis and the Critically Ill Patient.* Norwalk, CT: Appleton & Lange.

Roy, C., and Andrews, H. (1991). *The Roy Adaptation Model: The Definitive Statement.* Norwalk, CT: Appleton & Lange.

Stolte, K. (1989). Using health-oriented nursing diagnoses in medical-surgical nursing. *Journal of Advanced Medical Surgical Nursing, 1*(3), 73–82.

Table 12.1. Relationships Among Selected Wellness Nursing Diagnoses, Behaviors, and Interventions: Adults in Critical Care

Area	Wellness Nursing Diagnosis	Critically Ill Adult Behaviors	Nursing Interventions
Consciousness	*Maintaining consciousness and cognitive function*	Initiates use of supplemental oxygen for activities with increased metabolic demand	Leave equipment within reach
			Give positive feedback for appropriate independent use
		Negotiates pain medication dosage to promote pain relief without altering consciousness	Incorporate client desires into medication plan
	Maintaining effective communication	Asks questions about sounds and events occurring in the unit	Give brief explanations of unit activities, treatments, and procedures
		Asks for explanations about treatments and procedures	Ascertain understanding and clarify as necessary
		Uses paper and pencil, letter, board, gestures as alternative methods when unable to verbalize	Assist client to identify alternative methods to communicate

(continued)

Area	Wellness Nursing Diagnosis	Critically Ill Adult Behaviors	Nursing Interventions
Consciousness (cont'd.)	Maintaining effective communication (cont'd.)	Requests glasses and hearing aids as needed to communicate	Allow sufficient time for communication
			Assure aides are within patient's reach and in working order
Consistency of Behaviors	Progressing through the grieving process	Demonstrates behaviors consistent with movement from denial to anger and bargaining to acceptance/adaptation to loss	Provide safe environment for client to verbalize or act out feelings
			Assist client to channel aggression/anger/frustration constructively
		Incorporates client desires into mediation plan	
	Complying with the treatment plan	Takes medications as prescribed	Reinforce client's efforts to follow plan
		Follows suggestions of physician and nurse to prevent side effects	Collaborate with client to determine successful strategies and revise plan as needed
Characteristics of Client Background	Facilitating own emotional balance	Initiates own diversional activities such as reading, listening to	Encourage to identify diversional activities

	music, watching TV	Assure that items are within reach and in working order
		Facilitate acquisition of necessary items to support diversional activity
Acquiring knowledge	Asks for explanations about procedures and medications	Gives explanations as requested
		Offer information prior to procedures
Questioning care	Seeks additional information about disease process and interventions	Identify preferred learning mode and provide appropriate materials
Control of Movement *Improving activity tolerance*	Initiates increasing levels of activity, e.g., sitting in chair, ambulating in room	Support and monitor client's progress while increasing activity level
EMOTION Power *Retaining sense of control*	Actively seeks information	Provide opportunities to make decisions
	Participates in own care	

(continued)

Area	Wellness Nursing Diagnosis	Critically Ill Adult Behaviors	Nursing Interventions
EMOTION Power (cont'd.)	Retaining sense of control (cont'd.)	Makes decisions when given opportunity	Support client's decisions about medical care
Social Support	Maintaining social support networks	Expresses interest in understanding and participating in care	Provide opportunities for family to help with client care
			Provide familiar objects in client's room
	Maintaining family cohesiveness	Asks for family presence	Encourage family presence
			Promote flexible visiting policies
Self-Concept	Maintaining consistent self-concept	Applies positive coping strategies	Listen and support client
			Encourage positive coping
		Describes feelings of self-worth	Reinforce feelings of self-worth
Acceptance	Accepting limitations from illness/injury	Describes illness/injury in realistic terms	Reinforce realistic understanding of illness/injury
		Discusses ramifications of illness/injury	Explore meaning of illness event

		Discusses realistic changes in roles related to illness	Listen and support client
			Redirect avoidance behavior
			Clarify misunderstandings
			Begin teaching as readiness to learn is demonstrated
			Support efforts to maintain roles within realistic boundaries
Sensory Balance	*Maintaining sensory input balance*	Requests blocks of time with no interruption	Provide undisturbed rest periods
		Requests pain medicine before severe pain occurs	Reinforce behavior
		Discusses ways to limit noise and light	Offer alternative methods to control noise level such as white noise
			Provide consistent staff assignment
			Begin immediately to orient to unit

(continued)

201

Area	Wellness Nursing Diagnosis	Critically Ill Adult Behaviors	Nursing Interventions
Sensory Balance (cont'd.)	*Obtaining normal sensory input*	Wears sensory devices such as hearing aids and glasses	Address client using easily understood language
		Asks questions about environment	Encourage family interaction
			Encourage familiar objects in client's room
Sleep	*Maintaining usual sleep/rest cycle*	Requests periods of no interruption	Provide uninterrupted periods for sleep
		Discusses fear of sleep while recognizing need for sleep	Encourage familiar routines before sleep
			Help client identify fear (i.e., fear of not waking up)
PHYSIOLOGIC Cardiovascular: Regulatory Functions	*Progressive healing of myocardium*	Reduces physical activity	Affirm appropriateness of activity choices.
		Manages stress response	Assist client to meet ADL needs as necessary

	Client behaviors	Nursing interventions
		Support client's efforts to modify response to environment
Maintaining normal blood pressure during position changes	Sits on edge of bed prior to standing	Support client-initiated actions that prevent orthostatic hypotension
	Engages in active range of motion of lower extremities	
PULMONARY: Regulatory Functions		
Effective airway clearance	Uses incentive spirometer every 4 hours independently	Support use of spirometer by giving positive feedback for efforts and movement toward goal
	Increases inspired volume to meet goal	
Progressive weaning from the ventilator	Deliberately slows rapid breathing	Assists client to modify breathing pattern.
	Calls nurse for support when feeling anxious	Remain calm and give reassuring information about progress
	Attempts to steadily increase time off ventilator	Encourage client to extend time off ventilator

203

(continued)

Area	Wellness Nursing Diagnosis	Critically Ill Adult Behaviors	Nursing Interventions
PULMONARY: Regulatory Functions (cont'd.)	*Progressive weaning from the ventilator (cont'd.)*		Reinforce behavior
	Sustained ability to carry out self-care activities	Uses pursed-lip breathing to maximize expiration and prevent air-trapping	Reinforce use of breathing techniques
		Spaces activities so that energy is conserved	Assist client to establish activity/rest patterns
RENAL: Regulatory Functions	*Progressing toward fluid and electrolyte balance*	Negotiates fluid rationing throughout day	Reinforce appropriate sodium and fluid choices
		Substitutes hard candy for fluid if restricted	Assist client to identify alternate interventions to quench thirst
		Uses small quantity of ice for fluid volume	
		Maintains salt restriction	
GASTROIN-TESTINAL: Nutrition	*Progressing toward nutritional balance*	Steadily increases daily caloric intake	Facilitate alternative food choices by client and family

Skin Integrity	*Maintaining normal skin integrity*	Plans with dietitian and family members to eat desired high-caloric foods	Encourage family to provide client's favorite foods
		Adjusts frequency and amount of food intake to balance caloric needs and GI tolerance	Reinforce positive attempts to increase caloric intake
		Initiates position change routine	Incorporate client's suggestions for positioning
		Reports indicators of skin circulatory alteration such as erythema, numbness, etc.	Reinforce client's attentiveness of condition of skin
		Moves own paralyzed extremity	
Musculoskeletal	*Maintaining muscle strength*	Performs prescribed strengthening exercises	Reinforce behavior
			Assist client to set realistic goals and maintain sufficient work/rest routines
		Takes in sufficient calories to meet nutritional (especially protein) needs	Encourage protein intake.
			Assist client to obtain appropriate foods and supplements

13
~

Wellness Nursing Diagnoses in Home Health Care

With the impending changes in health care in the United States as well as the previous changes incurred with diagnosis-related groups (DRGs), the need for home health care is rapidly increasing. The Council on Scientific Affairs of the American Medical Association (1990) reports incorporation of home health care in medical school curricula and residency programs. In like fashion, nursing schools must evaluate the kinds of clinical experiences necessary to prepare nurses to help clients who need home care.

Many hospitals are reducing the number of beds, consolidating units, and cutting staff in order to cut costs. Hospital stays are reduced on all services and clients are returning to their homes or going to extended care facilities. In addition, a steadily growing elderly population creates a need to examine home health care resources for those who require assistance with activities of daily living and coping with chronic illness. The assumption that all people have someone at home who can help them with their care is erroneous. In many instances, an elderly spouse or partner may be unable to provide care for the other household member who is ill or recuperating from surgery. Because the number of single households is also increasing, the elderly are not the only clients who will need help at home.

Because of these trends, the acuity of clients being cared for in their homes or other community agencies has increased. Community health and home health nurses report they are now caring for clients who would have been hospitalized a few years ago. Using client strengths as a foundation for care will provide the client with hope, help the client focus on health rather than illness, and may facilitate the ability to cope with long-term illness.

~ Categories for Home Health Care Wellness Diagnoses

Saba (1992) devised a framework for classification and coding of diagnoses and interventions in home health care nursing that includes 20 different home health care components. Although the categories in this framework deal with impaired functioning or deficits, some of them can be modified or adapted for wellness behaviors and strengths.

A study by Thomas, Ellison, Howell, and Winters (1992) revealed that caregivers reported the following perceived needs of home health care clients receiving ventilatory support: social interaction with friends, participation in social activities outside the home, a daily routine, the ability to move from one room to another; and the ability to participate in self-care. These categories can be used to identify health-related behaviors.

~ Assessment of Strengths

The home health care client generally has many physical needs. Needs to maintain mobility, receive adequate nutrition, and maintain fluid and electrolyte balance, as well as needs specific to whatever disease process the client is experiencing, are often reasons for referral to home health care. No attempt will be made to deal with particular illnesses in this chapter, but some assessment areas specific to home health care clients will be addressed.

The reader is referred to the general strength assessment in Chapter 3 to find areas that apply to the home health care client. The wellness diagnoses found under nutrition, health-seeking behaviors, social support, spirituality, interaction with health care environment, compliance, and coping skills may all be relevant to the home health care setting.

Some of the wellness nursing diagnoses included in this chapter are identical to those in Chapter 3; others are more specific to the home health care client. Additionally, wellness nursing diagnoses identified in Chapter 11 for the older adult may apply to the home health care client.

Some components of Saba's (1992) framework have been adapted for use in this chapter. The following categories will be used to group the wellness nursing diagnoses considered for home health care: activity, health behavior, nutrition, fluid volume, role relationships, safety, and self-care. As in other chapters of this book, the wellness nursing diagnoses reflect client responses. The contributing factors (conditions) will be determined in the particular client situation.

Activity

The client who is able to maintain or regain as much mobility as possible will be able to achieve some degree of normalcy. If clients are mobile, they can participate in their care, enlarge their environment to include more than one room, and exert some control over their lifestyle.

Assessment of mobility can best be done by observation; however, the nurse may also consider the following assessment questions:

- How mobile is the client?
- What environmental factors facilitate or interfere with mobility?
- Is the client motivated to maintain mobility?
- What things does the client do to maintain or restore mobility?

Wellness nursing diagnoses related to mobility would include

~ *Maintaining current mobility*
~ *Progressive restoration of previous mobility status*

Health Behavior

Assessment of compliance of the home health care client falls under the category of health behavior. In addition, use of community resources that aid the client to obtain required care can be considered health behavior.

Clients receiving home health care are often under careful medical supervision that involves specific diets, medications, exercise regimens, etc. Compliance with these regimens is a major concern of the home health care nurse. However, before compliance can occur, the client often needs knowledge about why particular activities, drugs, treatments, and the like are prescribed. Although knowledge will increase the probability of compliance, it is not the only factor involved. Expectations that the prescribed regimen will be effective and acceptance of responsibility for self-care also influence the client's level of compliance. Assessment questions could include:

- How much knowledge does the client have about his or her treatment or disease process?
- Has the client actively sought information about his or her health care?
- What kind of expectations does the client have about treatment?
- Is the client willing to carry out his or her own self-care?
- How closely is the treatment regimen followed?

Wellness nursing diagnoses related to compliance include

~ *Actively seeking knowledge about medical treatment or disease process*
~ *Increasing acceptance of responsibility for self-care*
~ *Increasing compliance with prescribed treatment*

Home health care clients often need information about community resources and how to utilize them. The nurse can identify resources in the community that clients can use to further their care, including methods of transportation, resources for food and clothing, and financial assistance. In some instances, the client must take the initiative to obtain this assistance by completing the paperwork that proves eligibility for the service. Assessment questions related to this area might include:

- What does the client know about community resources that can be used to help carry out his or her care?
- What steps has the client taken to obtain information about these resources? To obtain their services?
- Is the client willing to use these resources?

A wellness nursing diagnosis would be

> ~ *Increasing utilization of community resources*

Nutrition

Maintenance of adequate nutrition and compliance with prescribed diet are issues in home health care. An adequate diet gives physical strength to cope with illness and provides nutrients for cognitive and immunological functioning. In addition, eating generally involves social interaction, which may provide stimulation for the client. Some assessment questions related to nutritional state are:

- What does the client know about nutrition?
- Does the client understand and follow the prescribed diet?
- If someone other than the client does meal preparation, does that person understand the diet and prepare appropriate meals?
- Is eating a social event in the home? If not, how can it become a social event?

Wellness nursing diagnoses related to these issues would be

> ~ *Increasing knowledge about adequate nutrition*
> ~ *Compliance with prescribed diet*
> ~ *Increasing social interaction while eating*

Fluid Volume

Fluid and electrolyte balance is a major concern in home health care. Imbalance may occur because of pathophysiological changes, medications, necessity for bed rest, or inadequate intake. Therefore, a proper balance reveals a client strength. Assessment questions might be:

- What does the client know about fluid needs?
- Does the client understand how medications influence electrolytes? Does the client know how to offset these changes? If so, what is the client's explanation?

Wellness nursing diagnoses related to this area would include

~ *Knowledge about prescribed fluid needs*
~ *Increasing knowledge about medication needs specific to fluid and electrolytes*

Role Relationships

Role relationships include social and spiritual needs and role change. Social interaction needs may be met by friends, participation in organizational activities if not totally home bound, or writing letters. Even though physically restricted, these clients may utilize community resources such as church outreach ministries or radio and TV programs to meet their spiritual needs. Assessment questions might include:

- What kind of social interaction does the client have?
- What can the client do to increase social interaction?
- What spiritual resources does the client have?
- Is the client aware of spiritual resources in the community and has he or she made use of them?

Clients who can mobilize their resources to meet social and spiritual needs could have the following wellness nursing diagnoses:

~ *Progressive social interaction*
~ *Actively seeking resources to meet spiritual needs*

Clients with acute or chronic disease often must undergo role changes due to limited physical ability, increased dependence on others, or changes in social relationships. Accommodation to these role changes may be difficult for the client who has always been active in home or community activities. However, clients often adjust to these changes by substituting one activity for another that more closely fits within their physical tolerance. Learning to accept help and maintaining control over those areas where it is feasible, while releasing control over those areas where it is not, are also behaviors that indicate adjustment to the new role. Assessment questions could include:

- How well has the client adapted to limitations?
- What alternative activities does the client describe that allow for interests to be maintained within physical limitations?
- Can the client let go of activities that are no longer possible?

A wellness nursing diagnosis would be

~ *Beginning acceptance of role change*

Safety

Providing home health care for a client may change the home environment in such a way that extra precautions must be taken to ensure safety. Use of medical technology (monitors, ventilators, and the like) necessitates consideration of electrical safety. Physical safety for the client includes proper use of side rails (if needed), well-balanced walkers or wheelchairs that can be locked in place, uncluttered walkways to bathrooms, and guardrails on stools or commodes that the client can grip to prevent falls. Medication safety includes clear labels, adequate lighting to read labels, appropriate prescriptive glasses, and a safe storage place. Assessment questions would include:

- How safe is the environment for the client?
- Is the client and/or caregiver aware of safety needs?
- What changes have been made to ensure a safe environment?

A wellness diagnosis related to safety would be

~ *Creating a safe environment conducive to health care*

Self-Care

Because many clients are moved from the hospital to their home for continuing health care while they are still in the acute stage of illness, they must deal with the transition from hospital to home. In general, clients see a hospital as a safe environment where they are protected by health care professionals and do not need to worry personally about their care. Leaving that safe environment may cause anxiety or fear.

Clients must start taking an active role in their own care if they have not done so in the hospital, and may need to find ways to alter their home environment to include space for equipment, supplies, etc. Not only do clients receiving home health care have to deal with new equipment or supplies at home, they may need to learn to use this equipment. For instance, the diabetic client must learn to use blood glucometers, give shots, etc. The first week at home is a prime time to evaluate the environment and help the client learn to carry out the prescribed medical regimen. Assessment questions could include:

- How does the client feel about receiving care at home?
- What ways can the client identify to give home care?
- How ready is the client to actively take part in his or her care?
- What kind of hospital instruction has the client received regarding his or her care?
- Does the client, or a family member, know how to handle equipment needed for care?

Wellness diagnoses related to this component would be

~ *Beginning transition to home care*
~ *Beginning skill in use of medical equipment/technology (specify)*

∼ *Wellness Nursing Diagnoses for the Caregiver*

In home health care the nurse must not only consider the client, but also work with the family and caregivers in order to provide care. Many articles have been written about the burden of the caregiver who has to provide continuous care to the home-bound client. The need for social support of the caregiver is found repeatedly in the literature (Thomas, Ellison, Howell, and Winters, 1992; Decker and Young, 1991). Hull (1993) identified the following coping strategies of caregivers in hospice home care: finding time to be relieved from caregiving; evaluating the situation in terms of other situations and finding positive aspects; minimizing stress by identifying benefits; taking an active role in caregiving in areas where it is possible to have control and giving up other areas; taking one day at a time; accepting the situation; and receiving social support.

When Thomas, Ellison, Howell, and Winters (1992) interviewed caregivers of persons receiving ventilatory support, they found the following personal needs: closeness among family members, care of own health; space for equipment; interaction with friends and family members; privacy and personal time; social support; social activities; and time away from home.

The nurse can encourage caregivers to focus on their particular strengths and can reinforce healthful behaviors that give the caregivers energy and resilience to cope with their situation. Behaviors reflecting that the above needs are met would be the basis for wellness nursing diagnoses.

Personal Needs

The caregiver who mobilizes resources in order to receive some relief from continuous caregiving would be demonstrating healthy behavior. During this release time, caregivers could talk to friends or family members and receive social support.

This personal time could also be used to meet personal needs for rest, since many caregivers do not get adequate sleep. Assessment of the caregiver might include these questions related to personal needs:

- Does the caregiver recognize the need for personal time?
- How much rest does the caregiver get?
- How does the caregiver find time for privacy and time to get personal errands done?
- How much time does the caregiver have away from the client?
- What alternatives for client care has the caregiver made in order to provide private time?

A wellness nursing diagnosis related to these activities would be

> ～ *Mobilizing efforts to meet personal/family needs*

Adjustment as a Caregiver

Another aspect of healthy caregiver behaviors is related to cognitive reformulation of perceptions, which enables the caregiver to deal with life one day at a time. Identifying benefits of having the client at home rather than in a hospital or nursing home, recognizing that others may be in worse situations than this one, and planning daily routines that deal with the present rather than anticipating the future are ways that caregivers cope (Hull, 1993). Assessment questions might include:

- How does the caregiver cope with demands?
- What value does the caregiver see to home care?
- What kind of lifestyle changes has the caregiver made?
- Are these changes realistic and feasible?
- How does the caregiver allow for flexibility in routine?

Wellness nursing diagnoses for these caregivers would be

> ～ *Beginning adjustment to caregiving status*
> ～ *Planning flexible routine for caregiving*

CASE STUDY

To illustrate the use of wellness nursing diagnoses in home health care, the following case study is presented. Jerry is a 45-year-old man with a diagnosis of AIDS. Over the course of the disease, he has had CMV (cytomegalovirus) and *Pneumocystis carinii* pneumonia. He is unable to work and has no health insurance. He is very weak and gets progressively weaker each day. His white blood cell counts, hemoglobin, and hematocrit are very low. At this point, he is unable to get out of bed without assistance. He has persistent nausea and is unable to eat anything except small amounts of pudding. Currently, he is in the terminal stages of the disease and is in a hospice program in a small town. Since the professional nurses donate their time, the hospice program is free except for the cost of home health aides.

In spite of his severe illness, Jerry maintains control over his environment and his health care. He wants to die at home and has refused tube feedings the hospice program would provide because he believes that those feedings would only prolong his life. He also says that if he started the tube feedings, he would not know when to stop them. The use of intravenous fluids would require hospitalization and he has refused them. Although home health care aides and professional nurses provide some of his care, he has also mobilized his friends who are willing to provide care for him. They have established a schedule that permits at least one friend to be there at all times. In addition, the friends have pooled their resources and are providing financial assistance to provide for drugs, the cost of the home health aides, and the costs of daily living. In order to maintain as normal a schedule as possible, he rises at the same time he did when he was working. Each day he requests that he be put in a recliner that is in front of a big window where he can see people go by. He has planned his funeral, prepared his will, and discussed his wishes with his friends. This ability to make plans, carry out his wishes, and prepare for his eventual death has given Jerry a sense of peace and he believes he can now die with dignity.

> Some wellness nursing diagnoses for Jerry are *increasing acceptance of responsibility for self-care*, *increasing utilization of community resources*, and *progressive social interaction*. Nursing interventions would be directed at facilitating his efforts to maintain control over his life and activities, mobilizing community resources to provide the needed care, and providing emotional support as the time for death approaches.

SUMMARY

In summary, a variety of wellness nursing diagnoses have been provided for use with the home health care client and caregiver. Tables 13.1 and 13.2 (see overleaf) illustrate the relationships among the wellness nursing diagnoses presented in this chapter, selected client/caregiver behaviors, and suggested interventions.

References

Council on Scientific Affairs (1990). Home care in the 1990s. *Journal of the American Medical Association, 263*(9), 1241–1244.

Decker, S.D., and Young, E. (1991). Self-perceived needs of primary caregivers of home-hospice clients. *Journal of Community Health Nursing, 8*(3), 147–154.

Hull, M.M. (1993). Coping strategies of family caregivers in hospice home care. *Caring, 12*(2), 78–88.

Saba. K. (1992). Diagnoses and interventions. *Caring, 11*(3), 50–57.

Thomas, V.M., Ellison, K., Howell, E.V., and Winters, K. (1992). Caring for the person receiving ventilatory support at home: Care givers' needs and involvement. *Heart and Lung, 21*(2), 180–186.

Table 13.1. Relationships Among Selected Wellness Nursing Diagnoses, Behaviors, and Interventions: Home Health Care Client

Wellness Nursing Diagnosis	Home Health Care Client Behaviors	Nursing Interventions
Maintaining current mobility	Range-of-motion, frequency and type of mobility patterns remain unchanged	Encourage mobility by suggesting activities appropriate to client ability
	Actively works on maintaining mobility by exercise regimen such as daily walking, working in yard, etc.	Reinforce exercise activities
		Perform range-of-motion exercises if needed and appropriate
Progressive restoration of previous mobility status	Actively participates in exercise regimen aimed at increasing activity level at increments appropriate for client ability	Explore activities that would aid in restoration to previous mobility state
		Reinforce participation in exercise regimen
	Suggests and implements alternative exercises as appropriate	Praise attempts at improvement or actual improvement
	Demonstrates improvement in mobility status	Carry out range-of-motion exercises or other exercise activities as appropriate

Actively seeking knowledge about medical treatment or disease process	Asks questions about treatment or disease process	Reinforce knowledge
	Seeks written material about treatment or disease process and reads it	Reinforce ability to ask health care professionals questions about treatment or disease process
	Describes relationships between disease process and treatment as appropriate	Provide information about treatment or disease process in oral, written, or audiovisual format
	Discusses activities specific to disease that will improve health	Discuss ways that client can improve health
Increasing acceptance of responsibility for self-care	Seeks information about health care/treatment	Recognize and reinforce idea that client is ultimately responsible for own care
	Discusses alternative ways to ensure that treatment regimen is followed	Explore alternative ways that treatment can be carried out within client's own particular lifestyle
	Actively decides the aspects of treatment for which he or she will assume responsibility	Support client decisions regarding continuing treatment or discontinuing treatment as appropriate
	May decide to refuse treatment and give reasons why	

219

(continued)

Wellness Nursing Diagnosis	Home Health Care Client Behaviors	Nursing Interventions
Increasing acceptance of responsibility for self-care (cont'd.)	Incorporates treatment regimen into daily lifestyle	
Increasing compliance with prescribed treatment	States purpose of treatment and explains treatment plan to be followed	Reinforce knowledge/compliant behaviors
	Follows treatment as prescribed—amount, time, method, etc., as appropriate	Answer questions or explain why treatment is needed
	Continues to seek/gain information about treatment	Discuss expectations of treatment and reinforce those that are realistic
	Adjusts lifestyle to fit treatment regimen	Support lifestyle changes that may be necessary to incorporate medical treatment into daily routine
	Discusses expectations of treatment	
Increasing utilization of community resources	Seeks information about community resources to meet health care needs	Provide information about community resources
	Lists community resources that could be used to meet health care needs	Explore pros and cons of these services with client

	Contacts community agencies or completes needed forms to obtain services	Aid in completion of forms, telephone contact, etc., as needed
Increasing knowledge about adequate nutrition	Describes daily intake that satisfies ADA minimum daily requirements	Reinforce knowledge
	Using a diet recall, reports a diet that is nutritionally sound	Clarify misunderstandings
		Give positive reinforcement for good nutritional behaviors
Compliance with prescribed diet	Describes prescribed diet	Clarify misunderstandings
	Able to make appropriate substitutions among allowed food items	Reinforce compliance
	Has appropriate food items in home	Identify ways to make diet more flexible
Increasing social interaction while eating	Identifies ways/times he or she can eat with family or friends	Suggest ways that meal preparation can be done simultaneously for family and client
	Incorporates prescribed diet into cooking for family as much as possible	Reinforce social activities while eating

(continued)

Wellness Nursing Diagnosis	Home Health Care Client Behaviors	Nursing Interventions
Increasing social interaction while eating (cont'd.)	Participates in conversation with family/friends during meal times	
Knowledge about prescribed fluid needs	Describes adequate fluid intake	Clarify misunderstandings
	From recall, demonstrates that fluid intake is adequate	Reinforce accurate knowledge
	Describes various ways to increase fluid intake as needed	Suggest ways that fluids can be increased or modified if needed
Increasing knowledge about medication needs specific to fluid and electrolytes	Describes accurate dosage and effects of medication on electrolytes and fluid balance	Reinforce knowledge and clarify misconceptions
	Describes reasons for medication	Reinforce compliance with medication regime
	Demonstrates that medication is taken accurately	
Progressive social interaction	Contacts friends and family by phone, letter, etc., as appropriate	Reinforce social interaction
	Initiates family activities	Suggest ways that social interaction can be initiated or maintained

	Participates in organizational, church, or other community activities within physical limitations	Suggest alternative social interaction if previous activities can no longer be carried out
Actively seeking resources to meet spiritual needs	If home bound, uses radio, church outreach programs, TV, Bible reading as resources for spiritual fulfillment	Provide information about community resources for home bound
	Displays religious objects as evidence of faith (rosary, Bible, religious pictures, etc.)	Reinforce spending time in meeting spiritual needs
	Sets time aside for devotional time/meditation	
Beginning acceptance of role change	Describes impact of illness on relationships with others	Encourage ventilation and expression of feelings
	Expresses feelings of loss	Provide empathic listening
	Discusses ways he or she can accommodate to illness by substituting other activities/hobbies/interests for those that must be given up	Explore alternatives to previous activities/hobbies/interests that fit within physical limitations
		Discuss ways to maintain control and ways to let go of control

(continued)

223

Wellness Nursing Diagnosis	Home Health Care Client Behaviors	Nursing Interventions
Beginning acceptance of role change (cont'd.)	Differentiates between those things that can be controlled and those that cannot	
	Lets go of those things that cannot be controlled	
Creating a safe environment conducive to health care	Identifies environmental hazards	Explore needs for safety
	Adjusts physical setting to allow space for equipment needed for care	Discuss ways to provide safe care
	Removes physical hazards, adds guardrails and safety devices as needed	Identify resources to obtain guardrails, needed equipment, etc.
		Reinforce recognition of need for safety
Beginning transition to home care	Discusses changes in the living space that must be made to accommodate treatment (space for supplies, medical equipment if needed, e.g., bed, monitors, IV equipment, etc.)	Discuss options in providing for space for equipment
		Explore alternatives for ways that care can be provided
	Discusses alternative ways to meet health care needs	Explore client's feelings about home health care as well as feelings about leaving the hospital while still ill

	Expresses feeling that care can be given in the home instead of the hospital	Mobilize community resources to meet client's health care needs
	Accepts health care professionals who enter the home to give care	Reinforce self-care activities
	Begins to take responsibility for own care	
Beginning skill in use of medical equipment/technology (specify)	States reason for the medical equipment/technology	Reinforce knowledge
	Describes correct use of the equipment/technology	Clarify misconceptions
	Lists advantages and/or disadvantages of equipment/technology	Demonstrate correct use of equipment/technology
	Demonstrates proper use of equipment/technology	Watch client use equipment/technology and reinforce accuracies while correcting mistakes
	Handles equipment with relative ease	

(continued)

225

Table 13.2. Relationships Among Selected Wellness Nursing Diagnoses, Behaviors, and Interventions: The Home Health Care Caregiver

Wellness Nursing Diagnosis	Home Health Care Caregiver Behaviors	Nursing Interventions
Mobilizing efforts to meet personal/family needs	Recognizes personal/family needs	Discuss personal and family needs
	Recognizes personal limitations	Explore ways to meet both client and family needs
	Seeks ways to obtain relief from caregiving in order to meet personal/family needs	Suggest community resources that will enable caregiver to get relief from caregiving
Beginning adjustment to caregiving status	Identifies benefits of having client at home	Explore positive and negative aspects of home health care and caregiving
	Incorporates client care into family life	Suggest ways to ease the burden of caregiving such as sharing among family members, etc.
	Compares own situation with others	
Planning flexible routine for caregiving	Considers alternative plans for routine caregiving	Explore caregiver and client needs
	Considers own needs while planning to meet client needs	Suggest alternative plans for routine care
	Plans routines with client input	Mobilize community resources to aid in routine care

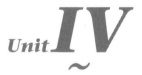

*W*ellness Nursing Diagnosis for Groups and Aggregates

~

14
~

Wellness Nursing Diagnoses for Groups

Community health nurses have traditionally identified clients as individuals, families, a group of persons working on a particular health issue, or communities. With the increasing concern for cost containment and the emphasis on health promotion, interest in aggregate groups of clients is escalating. The goals listed in *Healthy People 2000* (1990) are directed at particular segments of the population and reflect goals for the aggregate, not individual goals. The Pew Report (1991) also notes the need to prepare health professionals to work with groups in addition to individual clients.

Many opportunities exist for nurses to work with aggregates. These groups can be either hospital based or community based. For instance, psychiatric/mental health nurses work with psychotherapy groups, maternity nurses work with groups in prepared childbirth and parenting classes, and adult health nurses may work with groups of elderly clients in daily living centers.

What characteristics determine whether two or more individuals are a group or merely an aggregate of persons exhibiting similar personal or environmental characteristics? Many definitions exist in the literature. However, the essential characteristics for a group are interaction and interdependence among the group members. Without this interdependence, the group is merely a collective set of people. Nurses work with groups to help them accomplish some purpose related to health promotion or resolution of problems arising from illness.

In the following paragraphs, some aspects of group assessment are presented with examples of wellness nursing diagnoses from the literature. In addition, using the process approach discussed earlier, a few diagnoses are given for the reader to consider. As with the other chapters in this book, only the response portion of the diagnosis is included. The condition portion will vary with the particular situation.

When working with groups, as with individual clients, one must take into account the age, ethnicity, culture, geographical location, and religious preferences of the group. These factors will impact group performance, group cohesion, and group receptivity to intervention.

～ *Types of Groups*

Some types of groups that nurses may encounter in their practice are teaching–learning groups, support groups, and task-oriented groups. Teaching–learning groups are directed at helping clients learn how to incorporate specific lifestyle changes into everyday living. Groups for new diabetic clients, new cardiac clients, or new parents fall into this category. Interaction between group members is used to reinforce behaviors, gain new information, or share beneficial information gleaned from the group members' experiences.

Support groups encourage people to maintain the new behaviors they have learned or to prevent adoption of behaviors that are not useful. Discussion of feelings helps group members learn that they are not alone and helps them recognize that new behaviors can be developed that last over time. Recognition of client strengths in these groups serves to reassure clients and to reinforce the idea that they will succeed in meeting the crisis or making the required changes.

Task-oriented groups usually entail problem solving or collaborative endeavors. These groups are formed to carry out a specific function during a particular time frame. Once the task is accomplished, the group disbands.

~ Group Tasks and Group Maintenance

The ability to work with groups is quite different from one-to-one interactions. It must be remembered that a group response is more than the sum of the individual responses. This perspective is quite complex.

When working with a group, awareness is needed of both the task of the group as well as group process or the way the group members interact with each other. Group maintenance involves the way that the group works together to accomplish its task. The ease in which group tasks are achieved depends on how carefully group maintenance is preserved. Maintenance functions are directed toward helping the individuals in the group feel accepted or supported. Avoidance of conflict or resolution of conflict are also maintenance functions.

Group task functions relate to the goal of the group and facilitate goal achievement. Ability to problem solve, suggest resources, or focus the group on the topic are skills related to group member tasks.

A balance between task functions and maintenance functions must be maintained. If the leader, generally the nurse, attends only to maintenance functions, the task may never be completed. If attention is only given to the task at hand, group members may feel isolated and unappreciated, and the ability to carry out the task is impeded.

~ Pattern of Group Process

The group process follows a general pattern. Initially, the group attempts to become a group rather than a number of individuals. They are dependent on the leader to tell them what to do and seek structure and organization for the group.

As the interaction continues, control issues emerge with some members trying to take control of the group, which results in group conflict. During this phase, the leader's authority is questioned and often diminishes as other leaders emerge. The group as a whole must work out these conflicts. Using open communication, the members will ultimately arrive at the next stage of group development where they recognize their interdependence. At this point, the task can be completed with each member believing that he or she made a contribution and expressing satisfaction with group accomplishments.

The nurse who leads a group must have knowledge about group process as well as knowledge about the specific content to be discussed in the group. Often two nurses will lead a group in order to be sure that both task and maintenance behaviors are supported. Assessment of the group involves determination of the stage of group work as well as the content to be covered in a particular group session if it is a teaching–learning group.

~ Assessment of Group Strengths

Allen (1993) points out that not all group nursing diagnoses need to be illness oriented. Identification of group members' strengths and positive responses to particular health-related conditions can provide the foundation for group wellness nursing diagnoses. In groups where content is included, such as teaching–learning groups, wellness nursing diagnoses may be content-focused diagnoses or group process–focused diagnoses. In those instances, the first-level assessment involves the content. A second-level assessment relates to group process.

Most information in the literature about group diagnoses relates to either the family or community. A few articles were found about groups per se, but no specific wellness diagnoses were included. Remembering that assessment must culminate in finding commonalities among the members, data can be obtained that will support adapting some individual diagnoses to group situations, resulting in group diagnoses. There are diagnoses presented in Chapters 3, 4, and 9 of this book that can be adapted to groups. Most of these deal with content issues. Examples from Chapter 3 are

~ *Increasing knowledge about adequate nutrition*
~ *Increasing ability to avoid stressful situations*
~ *Beginning practice of stress management techniques*
~ *Progressive identification and elimination of negative health care practices*
~ *Actively seeking knowledge about medical treatment or disease process*
~ *Beginning preparation for maturational/developmental event*
~ *Seeking interaction with others to learn new skill/role*
~ *Increasing compliance with prescribed treatment*

Examples from Chapter 9 include

~ *Increased problem-solving ability*
~ *Beginning acceptance of parenting role*
~ *Reevaluating and developing parenting skills consistent with growing children*

Diagnoses found in Chapter 4 that can be applied to prepared childbirth groups include

~ *Beginning acceptance of reality of pregnancy*
~ *Progressive preparation for labor*

No doubt the reader could identify other diagnoses in those chapters that would also be relevant for groups.

Assessment of the maintenance ability of a group results in wellness nursing diagnoses related to group maintenance and group process. To assess group process and group maintenance the nurse might consider the following assessment questions:

■ Who is the group leader?
■ Who are the informal leaders as well as the formal leaders?
■ How cohesive is the group?

- What kind of norms has the group developed?
- What are the expectations of group members?
- Do all group members participate in group discussions? If so, how?
- How do group members support and reinforce each other?
- If appropriate, do group members share feelings as well as information? If so, in what ways?

The group who has developed a set of norms that are consistently followed through both verbal and nonverbal communication would have this wellness diagnosis:

~ *Continued consistency of group norms*

A group in which each member participates actively, contributes to the group discussion or problem-solving process, and provides encouragement to other group members could have a wellness diagnosis of

~ *Progressive group interdependence*

A teaching–learning group that enables group members to share feelings and provides reinforcement for both the sharing and the feelings themselves would have a wellness diagnosis of

~ *Increasingly supportive group climate*

CASE STUDY

Mary Smith, R.N., facilitates a teaching–learning group on parenting. Mary and eight clients meet 1 hour once a week to discuss parenting skills as well as to identify ways to reduce the stress involved with being parents of new infants. When they enrolled for the group, these clients told Mary that they wanted to learn more about parenting and the developmental changes in children during the first 2 years of life.

Initially, Mary presented several ideas to the group about topics that might be discussed. Over time, a general format for each group session has evolved that includes a short formal presentation about a specific topic such as play activities, providing a safe environment, realistic expectations of specific age groups, or setting limits. The group members then talk about whatever parenting concerns or questions they have that particular week.

Because they have been meeting for approximately 6 weeks, the group members now participate freely. Mary has seen progression in the group's ability to share their feelings openly and to talk about their own experiences in dealing with particular concerns that are expressed by others. Those group members who are first-time parents often ask those who have several children to explain how they handled specific problems. Mary has noticed that many of the group members now praise each other for their input. They also express gratitude for possible solutions that are suggested for problems. The group frequently discusses the pros and cons of the solutions that are offered.

In addition, the group members take responsibility to point out if someone monopolizes the conversation. Therefore, the group members are active participants who can focus on both group task and group maintenance activities. Group-focused wellness nursing diagnoses for this group might be *increasingly supportive group climate, continued consistency of group norms,* and *progressive group interdependence.* A content-focused wellness nursing diagnosis might be *increasing knowledge about parenting skills* or *increasing ability to problem solve.*

SUMMARY

This chapter has focused on wellness diagnoses for groups. Current changes in health care predict that nurses will work more with groups than with individual clients. Although in its infancy, the need for aggregate diagnoses will increase. The complexity of assessment and diagnosis rises exponentially as the number of persons who make up the client base increases. Although the discipline of nursing has not developed as many problem-oriented diagnoses for groups as for individuals, even fewer wellness diagnoses exist. Based on assessment criteria for healthy group interaction, some wellness diagnoses have been proposed. Examples of the relationships among wellness diagnoses, behaviors, and interventions for groups are presented in Table 14.1.

References

Allen, M.E. (1993). Mental health. In J.M. Swanson and M. Albrecht (eds.), *Community Health Nursing: Promoting the Health of Aggregates* (pp. 487–503). Philadelphia: Saunders.

Healthy People 2000: National Health Promotion and Disease Prevention Objectives (1990). Washington, DC: United States Department of Health and Human Services, USPHS.

Sugars, D.A., O'Neil, G.H., Bader, J.D. (eds.) (1991). *Healthy America: Practitioners for 2005, an Agenda for Action for US Health Professional Schools*. Durham, NC: The Pew Health Professions Commission.

Table 14.1. Relationships Among Selected Wellness Nursing Diagnoses, Behaviors, and Interventions: Groups

Wellness Nursing Diagnosis	Group Behaviors	Nursing Interventions
Continued consistency of group norms	Group members can state group norms	Facilitate development of group norms
	Group members point out any behaviors inconsistent with group norms when they occur	Praise group for development and follow-through of group norms
	If necessary, group norms are modified through group process	Remind members of group norms if deviation occurs
Progressive group interdependence	Group members are aware that they cannot function independently from the group	Remind group of task to be achieved
	Each group member actively contributes to group task either verbally or nonverbally	Reinforce group behaviors directed toward group task
	Group discussion is focused on needs of the group rather than individual members	Encourage participation of individual group members
		Reinforce group rather than individual activities

(continued)

237

Wellness Nursing Diagnosis	Group Behaviors	Nursing Interventions
Increasingly supportive group climate	Group members encourage each other to share feelings and/or ideas	Encourage openness and spontaneity
	Group members reinforce each other's participation	Encourage sharing of feelings and/or ideas
	Group members are treated with respect and recognized as equals	Praise and reinforce group members' respect of each other

15
~

Wellness Nursing Diagnoses for Families

As mentioned in Chapter 14, the increasing concern for cost containment and the emphasis on health promotion has created a growing interest in aggregate groups. One group that is becoming more and more important in nursing practice is the family. Incorporation of the family into nursing care has been a major activity in pediatric and maternity nursing for years. Community health nurses have long been aware of the importance of determining what kinds of health needs exist in a household. Inclusion of family members in inpatient and outpatient nursing care is increasing.

In this heterogeneous society, many types of family units exist. No longer is the typical family composed of a father, mother, and children. Although nuclear families are probably more common than extended families in our mobile society, many types of families exist including blended families consisting of parents and children from current and previous marriages, one-parent families, cohabitating families, and cross-cultural families. In addition, adults who live together but are not related by blood may make up a family. Caudle and Grover (1992) define a family as "a social system composed of two or more people living together who may be related by blood, marriage, or adoption, or who stay together by mutual agreement" (p. 396).

Working with a family unit is much more complex than working with individual clients. Family interaction patterns are influenced by the family structure, the stage of life-cycle development, and family functioning. The family has a major impact on how well the individual deals with health and illness. One of the tasks of the family is to secure health care for family members. Culture, ethnicity, local customs, and religious beliefs all play a part in the type of health care sought by the family and the compliance that is given to the recommendations made by health care providers.

∼ Wellness Family Nursing Diagnoses in the Literature

Currently NANDA has one wellness family diagnosis: *Family Coping: Potential for Growth* (NANDA, 1994, p. 54). The NANDA diagnosis *Altered Family Processes* (NANDA, 1994, p. 43) might be used as a wellness diagnosis except the defining characteristics lead one to believe that positive functioning is threatened by a stressor, so the focus is not exactly on wellness. Using NANDA diagnoses, Ross and Cobb (1990) describe two family diagnoses: "*Family Coping, Potential for Growth, related to willingness of family to seek assistance in planning and decision making* and *Health Seeking Behaviors, related to recognition of couple's nutrition needs, desire to lose weight and to improve nutritional intake for Mrs. J.*" (p. 68). No other wellness diagnoses for families were found.

∼ Characteristics of a Healthy Family

Who is the healthy family? In discussing health promotion for the well family, Petze (1984) notes that family models have changed over time from authoritarian male-dominated models to more egalitarian models that focus on mutual goals, responsibility for growth and development of each member, and provision of material goods. The family as a unit is responsible for helping each family member develop to his or her full potential, assisting in attainment of both individual and family goals, and fostering autonomy and flexibility among its members.

The family serves a protective function for its members. It provides support, socializes children, meets basic needs of food and shelter, and is a "safe" place from the outside world. As a part of society, the family is a subsystem of a larger social system.

Petze (1984) describes family competencies as "communication skills, previous learning and associated coping behaviors, insight into one's own actions and motivations, ability to connect with others emotionally, ability to be honest and open in dealings with others, problem solving capacity and follow through on plans" (p. 231). The healthy traits of a single-parent family are "functional communication, adequate social support, spiritual orientation and good decision making patterns" (Bomar, 1990, p. 2).

It is essential to note that every family has strengths and weaknesses. Since the focus of this book is on wellness diagnoses, family strengths will be emphasized in this chapter. Most authors suggest that family assessment begin with identification of family strengths. Involving the family in identification of its strengths starts the nurse–client relationship on a positive note and gives the family tools that can be used to offset weaknesses. In addition, this recognition of strengths makes them more amenable to identification of problems or weaknesses and to intervention.

Family strengths are the cornerstone that help the family cope with times of transition and change. Curran (1985) notes that the family who can cope with stress is one who views stress as a normal event, knows how to be creative, has conflict resolution skills, can adapt, shares feelings, and uses its support systems effectively. In addition, Smilkstein (1984) states that the healthy family is described by its members as cohesive. It offers physical and emotional resources that promote the growth and development of family members.

Family hardiness characterizes a family who actively works together to solve problems, has a sense of control over outcomes, and views change as beneficial (McCubbin, 1993). Families who have this group of characteristics are more able to cope with problems than families who do not. Curran (1983) also identifies traits of the healthy family (see Display 15.1).

In summary, common threads in the literature on healthy families seem to be open communication, an environment that nurtures and sustains individual family members as well as the family unit, clear yet flexible definition of roles, and ability to express warmth, intimacy, and humor. These families enjoy being together and are committed to each other. In addition, they interact with the society around them. In terms

DISPLAY 15.1.
Traits of the Healthy Family

1. Communicates and listens
2. Affirms and supports one another
3. Teaches respect for others
4. Develops a sense of trust
5. Has a sense of play and humor
6. Exhibits a sense of shared responsibility
7. Teaches a sense of right and wrong
8. Has a strong sense of family in which rituals and traditions abound
9. Has a balance of interaction among members
10. Has a shared religious core
11. Respects the privacy of one another
12. Values service to others
13. Fosters family table time and conversation
14. Shares leisure time
15. Admits to and seeks help from others

Source: Curran, 1983, pp. 23–24.

of health, these families have positive health practices both
as individuals and as a group.

Wellness nursing diagnoses that would reflect the family
strengths described in the preceding paragraphs would be

~ *Progressive sharing by family members of thoughts, per-*
  ceptions, and feelings
~ *Continued mutual problem solving which recognizes indi-*
  vidual and family needs
~ *Progressive flexibility in identification and allocation of*
  family members' responsibilities
~ *Mutual love and respect for all family members*

~ Assessment of Family Strengths

Since complete assessment of families is beyond the scope of
this book, the reader is referred to books on family nursing or
family assessment for further information. In the following
paragraphs, some aspects of family assessment are presented
with examples of wellness nursing diagnoses from the literature as well as those developed by the author. As with the
other chapters in this book, only the response portion of the
diagnosis is included. The condition portion will vary with the
particular situation.

The Nurse and the Family

A good beginning for assessment is to ask what health means
to the family. How does their definition of health fit into their
value system? Some families believe that if they can get up
every morning and do their work, they are healthy. They are
not concerned with health promotion and, in fact, may be living with some health problems for which they have not sought
treatment. Economic realities, lack of health insurance, or
lack of other resources such as transportation have made it
necessary for them to do the best with what they have. Health
screening or primary health prevention have a low position
in their value system because this care cannot be obtained

without using resources that must be distributed elsewhere.

When reading the literature about well families, characteristics are presented that are typically white, middle- or upper-class values. Although little is written about other types of families, Lynch and Tiedje (1991) clearly delineate some of the differences in family structure, communication processes, and socialization of children between the multiproblem family and the "typical" middle-class family. In general, multiproblem families do not have routine patterns, communicate to exhibit power rather than exchange ideas, and are concrete thinkers who do not deal with abstract ideas well. Nevertheless, these families can have strengths that must be fostered in order to help them cope with their immediate problems.

Lynch and Tiedje (1991) also describe some of the differences in values and use of information between the family and the health care provider. The family and the health care provider may become involved in a struggle over control. The authors declare that it is important for the nurse to leave the control with the family, ask for their suggestions when problem solving, and request permission to give information rather than dispense information without any consideration of situation or feelings. Just as with the individual, mutual goal setting with the family and nurse is essential for success to occur. In order to reach mutual goals, the nurse must meet with all family members as a group, not with one family member who will speak for the family or with individual family members at separate times.

Methods of Family Assessment

When reviewing the literature, some common methods of family assessment emerge: assessment of family function and structure; assessment of the family using a systems approach; a developmental approach to family assessment; and a functional health patterns approach using Gordon's (1994) functional health patterns. Many assessment guides are available in textbooks and other published material.

The nursing models have also been examined to determine how useful they are in dealing with families rather than individuals. Most of the models can be modified in some way to include the family; however, Neuman's (1995) model seems to be the one most frequently used for the family. These models can provide another framework for assessment.

Thomas, Barnard, and Sumner (1993) list five areas for family assessment from which wellness diagnoses can be derived: family processes, family coping, parenting, health maintenance and management, and home maintenance and management. They also provide a list of assessment tools for each area.

Although any of the family assessment methods can be used to develop wellness nursing diagnoses, two examples of family assessment methods will be presented. Exclusion of the other methods of family assessment does not mean that wellness diagnoses are not appropriate, but space limitations do not allow for listing every possible method. It is possible that some of these diagnoses could be used with other methods of assessment as well.

Family Functional Health Patterns Framework for Wellness Diagnoses

One method of family assessment involves use of Gordon's functional health patterns to determine the health practice patterns of a family (see Display 15.2). Some examples of questions that might be asked when assessing these patterns are given in the following paragraphs. These questions are adapted from Ross and Cobb (1990), who also pose additional questions not included here. Nettle, Pavelich, Jones, and Beltz (1993) also describe using this method of family assessment.

Health Perception/Health Management Pattern

- How does the family define health?
- Does the family perceive itself as healthy?
- What kinds of health practices do they have?

- How do they manage their health?
- What do they do when someone is ill?

Nutritional/Metabolic Pattern

- What are the family's nutritional patterns?
- What kinds of food do they eat and how often?
- How often do family members eat together?
- Do they know how to shop within the limits of their financial ability to get the most nutritious foods?
- How do they describe good nutrition?

Elimination Pattern

- What kind of hygiene do family members practice?
- How do they dispose of trash?

Activity/Exercise Pattern

- What kinds of activities does the family do together?
- How do they choose activities?
- In what ways do they get regular exercise?

DISPLAY 15.2.

Gordon's Functional Health Patterns

1. Health perception/health management pattern
2. Nutritional/metabolic pattern
3. Elimination pattern
4. Activity/exercise pattern
5. Cognitive/perceptual pattern
6. Sleep/rest pattern
7. Self-perception/self-concept pattern
8. Role/relationship pattern
9. Sexuality/reproductive pattern
10. Coping/stress tolerance pattern
11. Value/belief pattern

Source: Gordon, 1994, p. 70.

Sleep/Rest Pattern

- Where do family members sleep?
- How much sleep do they get?
- Do younger members have a chance to rest in the day-time?
- Do they get up early, stay up late, etc?
- How is the environment conducive to sleep?

Cognitive/Perceptual Pattern

- How does the family reach a decision?
- How do they deal with conflict?
- How do they approach a problem that needs to be solved?

Self-Perception/Self-Concept Pattern

- How do the individual members feel about the family as a unit?
- How do they reach out to the community when they need help?
- How do they think others view them as a family unit?

Role/Relationship Pattern

- How do family members support each other?
- What opportunities are there for the family members to interact with each other?
- What kind of role does each family member have?
- Are they satisfied with these roles?

Sexuality/Reproductive pattern

- Are sexual relationships fulfilling?
- How are children given age-appropriate sex education?
- What are the reproductive patterns in the family—spacing of children, use of birth control methods, health state during pregnancy, etc.?

Coping/Stress Tolerance Pattern

- What kind of crises have they experienced and what did they do to cope with the stress?

- What stress management techniques do they practice?
- Do they ask for help when they can no longer cope?

Value/Belief Pattern

- What does the family say they want to accomplish?
- What religious, spiritual, or cultural beliefs do they have that guide their purpose in life?
- How are they teaching their children these beliefs?
- How do these beliefs influence their health practices?

In terms of wellness nursing diagnoses related to these functional health patterns, several possibilities exist. If the nurse determines that the family is working on improving its patterns so the family will have better nutrition, more rest, increased activity, etc., the diagnosis would be

~ *Progressive improvement of (name of pattern)*

Family Developmental Tasks Framework for Wellness Diagnoses

The following paragraphs describe wellness diagnoses related to family developmental tasks. The information presented here is not intended to deal with every developmental task or with all possibilities for wellness diagnoses.

Duvall and Miller (1985) list an eight-stage family life cycle. The stages include beginning families; childbearing families; families with preschool children; families with school children; families with teenagers; families launching young adults; middle-aged families; and aging families. Although identification of the family's primary stage of development is determined by the age of the oldest child, the family may be in several stages at the same time depending on the ages of the children.

It is essential to remember that within these family developmental stages, individual family members are proceeding through various developmental tasks that the family must also foster. Also within these developmental tasks, the family must maintain the primary functions of socialization, provision of health care, reproduction, and economic stability. The reader can begin to see how complex assessment of the family becomes if all these elements are taken into account.

The following paragraphs are limited to family developmental tasks of a nuclear family. Accommodation to various types of families and various cultural groups will be needed. Although the original work on family developmental tasks is by Duvall (1977) and Duvall and Miller (1985), the source of much of the following information is Friedman and Miller (1992). The reader is referred to Friedman and Miller for a discussion of the developmental tasks of the divorced family and the remarried family.

Beginning Families   The beginning family occurs as the couple establishes a home after marriage or after a couple has made a commitment to each other to live together. Developmental tasks relate to establishing a mutually satisfying relationship, planning a family, and establishing ties to extended family members or kinship networks. The couple must learn ways to deal with conflict, consider different ways of doing things, and establish an identity of the family as a unit rather than identifying with parents or previous relationships. Attachment bonds that provide mutual support and encouragement must be solidified.

Initially, the couple must develop patterns of living for their household. Patterns of eating and sleeping, division of labor to accomplish household chores, use of leisure time, and budget management must be negotiated. Some assessment questions the nurse might consider for the beginning family include:

- What goals does the couple have?
- What does the couple enjoy doing together?
- Is the couple able to share thoughts and feelings openly?
- How does the couple handle conflict?
- What adjustments has each person made in order to develop a pattern of living that is acceptable to both of them?

- What patterns of living have emerged?
- Are individual as well as family needs being met?
- How much does the couple rely on extended family members for decision making, financial arrangements, etc.?
- What kind of emotional ties does the couple have with their extended family?

Wellness nursing diagnoses for the beginning family could include

~ *Progressive development of mutually satisfying relationship*
~ *Beginning development of the family unit*
~ *Developing ties to extended family*

Childbearing Families   The childbearing family begins with the birth of the first child and ends when that child is 2 $1/2$ years old. Integration of the new baby into the family is a major task as well as making the transition to parenthood. The wellness diagnoses cited in Chapter 4 that deal with the childbearing family are related to this stage of family development. Although written with one or either parent in mind, they can be modified to fit the family unit.

The addition of a child to a family necessitates changes in parents' roles toward each other. Couples see each other in a new light—that of parent as well as lover. The couple must find a way to meet their adult needs as well as those of the child. Time for intimacy, sexual fulfillment, and sharing is crucial. In order to assimilate these new roles, as well as, meet their own needs, couples must find time alone for discussion, sharing, and intimacy. As the child grows, the parents must accommodate to this growth, recognizing the autonomy that is developing in the child, and rearranging the environment to fit the child's needs. Relationships with friends, parents, and other family members also change as a result of the new baby. Conflict between generations over different ways to raise a baby may occur and must be resolved. For working parents, the balancing of multiple roles may become paramount to family harmony.

Couples must develop their own child care techniques,

methods of discipline, and child care patterns. Although they may receive input from parents, professionals, and others, ultimately they must assume responsibility for the infant's care and find child care methods that are acceptable and comfortable for them. The infant's mother often assumes total care and becomes the gatekeeper who regulates how much contact the father has with the infant. Mutually satisfying decisions must be made about how often, and from whom, the infant receives care. Accommodations must be made for the different ways men handle infants than women. Respect and confidence in each other is necessary. Some assessment questions for the childbearing family are:

- What time does the couple find for intimacy?
- How does the couple fine time to be alone without the baby?
- Are they able to leave the baby with others without feeling guilty?
- How does each family member view the other? As a parent? As a lover?
- How has their relationship with extended family members, friends, and others changed since the birth of the baby?
- What patterns of child care have they adopted?
- Are they each confident in caring for the child? Are they confident about each other's ability to care for the child? Can they relinquish child care to the other if needed?

Wellness nursing diagnoses that could be used with the childbearing family include

~ *Increasing allocation by couple of time alone without the infant*

~ *Progressive development of family child care patterns*

Families with Preschool Children   This stage begins when the first child is 2 1/2 and ends at the age of 5. Since one of the main functions of the family is to socialize its children, this task takes on new meaning. As the family unit enlarges, it becomes more complex. Not all the needs of the family can be met within the walls of the home. Children must have opportunities to play and interact with other children their own age in a variety of settings such as zoos, preschools, and parks. Therefore, family activities must encompass some of these activities and settings. Each member of the family must be respected regardless of age in order to develop his or her full potential.

A fine balance exists in order to attend to both children's and parents' needs. As new children are added to the family, they must be integrated in such a way that older children are not threatened and still have their needs met. Allocation of time alone with older children will help them realize that they are not being replaced by the new infant. Just as parents learn new roles as the family size increases and children grow, older children also learn new roles.

Continued relationships with extended family members and friends must be preserved as the family grows. Care must also be taken to ensure that the couple's relationship is maintained. Parents need outside interests as well as home responsibilities to help them lead balanced lives. This balance may be difficult in one-parent families since there is little time or money to pursue interest or hobbies.

Depending on the number and ages of children, family resources may be strained in order to meet the needs for housing, food, and clothing. This strain is particularly true for one-parent families. Ability to find additional resources within constraints of the family budget, such as trading children's clothing among extended family members or buying clothing at garage sales, is a strength. Use of community agencies to increase resources if necessary is also a strength. Assessment questions related to the family with preschool children could include:

- How do parents build time for themselves as a couple into their schedule?
- In what kinds of activities does the family engage?
- What is the parents' level of understanding of normal growth and development? In what ways do they provide age-appropriate activities for their children?
- How do the parents interact with their children?

- As children get older, do they participate in family discussions?
- Do the parents spend some time alone with each individual child?
- As family size increases, how do roles for each family member change?
- What kinds of resources does the family have?
- If needed, does the family know community resources that can be used to help augment family resources?

The following wellness diagnoses would be useful for the family with preschool children:

~ *Increasing social interaction appropriate for children's ages and abilities*

~ *Progressive inclusion of children in family discussions and decisions*

~ *Adapting individual roles within the family to accommodate changes in family configuration or size*

~ *Increasing utilization of family and community resources*

~ *Increasing ability of individual family members to give and take in order to meet each other's needs*

Families with School-Age Children   This stage begins when the eldest child is 6 and continues until the child reaches adolescence at age 13. Children's involvement in school, even if they have attended preschool, evokes changes in family life. Children begin to have more outside activities, transportation is often necessary to attend these activities, and parents often feel like they are taxicabs driving from place to place, especially when several children become school age. Focus on children's academic success may occur as well as helping children maintain peer relationships after school or on weekends. As a child matures, parents must alter their parenting techniques to allow for the child's growth and development. The time for letting go in accord with the child's ability is at hand. As with the previous stages, the task of maintaining a satisfying marital relationship continues. Assessment questions for the family with school-age children could include:

- How have parenting techniques been altered with the children's growth?
- Do the parents allow time for themselves?
- How does the family accommodate increased needs for transportation, varying schedules of family members, and academic needs of children?

Since methods of parenting must be modified to accommodate the increased independence and responsibility of the children, this diagnosis, discussed in Chapter 9, would be appropriate for this developmental stage:

> ~ *Reevaluating and developing parenting skills consistent with needs of growing children*

Families with Teenagers   This stage brings many new challenges to the family unit. The length varies depending on the age of the oldest child when he or she leaves the family home. A delicate balance between helping the teenager establish responsibility within the bounds of freedom must be developed and maintained. As the child becomes increasingly independent, the parents must alter their parenting styles.

Additionally, a shift in the parent–child relationship occurs as the child matures and prepares to leave home. No matter how much parents have worked to develop close communication with their children, some conflict will occur as the child strives for autonomy. Since teenagers often question their parents' values, parents will find these values tested and must remain firm. Assessment questions could include:

- How does the family cope with the normal conflict that arises when a teenager is in the family?
- How have parenting techniques been altered to incorporate more freedom for the teenager?
- Has the family been able to maintain open communication in the midst of conflicting values? If so, in what ways?

Wellness diagnoses for the family with teenagers could be

> ~ *Maintaining balance between independent and dependent needs of children*

~ *Continued commitment to family values*

Families Launching Young Adults This stage starts when the first child leaves home and is finished when the last child leaves home. Due to difficult economic times in our society, children often return to the "nest," so the length of time it remains "empty" may vary from family to family. If children come and go, it may be difficult to achieve family developmental tasks. Conflict may occur if children have been on their own and then return to their parents' home. Role relationships often become confused, creating the need to maintain open communication.

As children leave home, the couple must change the focus of their relationship as well as develop new roles, since the primary parenting role no longer exists. A woman who has never worked must find new interests. Both parents may realize that the dreams they once had will never be accomplished and adjustments must be made in expectations. They have more time alone and may need to relearn how to use this time. Spending more time together, exploring each other's interests, and sharing common concerns and goals will help the couple shift the emphasis from children back to the original couple.

As children marry, changes occur in the extended family and these new family members must be incorporated into the family unit. An appropriate diagnosis is

~ *Integration of new family member*

Assessment questions for this family development stage could include:

- If children have returned home, how has the family dealt with changing roles?
- What activities are parents involved in now that their children have left home?
- How has the couple adapted to being a two-member family again?
- What expectations do the parents have for themselves?

A wellness diagnosis could be

~ *Beginning reestablishment of a mutually satisfying couple relationship*

Middle-Aged Families   This stage starts when the last child leaves home and continues until one parent retires or dies. The need for companionship and leisure activities that both members of the couple can enjoy are major driving forces. The original couple also has to attain some kind of balance in terms of independence and dependence on each other. They may have a number of independent activities due to different interests, yet recognize their dependence on each other for companionship and mutual support.

With aging, the couple must deal with health concerns and find ways to maintain or improve their health. Changes in lifestyle may be needed in order to adapt to physical limitations. Relationships with grown children and the previous generation need to be sustained. The entry of grandchildren into the extended family also changes role relationships. Many of the wellness diagnoses in Chapter 10 related to the person in middle adulthood can be modified for the middle-aged family. Assessment questions might include:

- How does the couple find a balance between personal interests and mutual interests?
- What type of emotional support do they provide each other?
- How are they adapting to minor health changes?
- Since their children's families are now part of their extended family, what kind of relationship do they have with these family members?

A wellness diagnosis for this stage of family development might be

~ *Progressive reestablishment of a mutually satisfying couple relationship*

Aging Family This stage begins with retirement of one or both of the spouses and continues until death. Role adjustment occurs after retirement and the couple has to find satisfying alternatives to work. Many older persons gain fulfillment from helping others. If they are healthy and physically active, and reach out to others, this time of life is often rewarding. They can look back with pride on their accomplishments and do some of the things they planned, but never had the time, to do. As a family unit, the couple may choose to be involved in community activities.

Continued satisfaction is gained from the marital relationship. With aging, social relationships often decrease. Therefore, social support from the extended family becomes very important. Ties to the extended family, i.e., children, grandchildren, and siblings, need to be maintained.

Frequently these partners review their life experiences and spend time reminiscing. Such time is well spent as it helps the couple make sense of life, provides insight, and helps adjustment to difficult situations.

Lastly, many losses occur during this time, but the family can and usually will adjust to these losses as a part of normal life transitions. Examples of these losses include loss of income, loss of a spouse, and loss of friends. Alternative housing arrangements may need to be explored. Assessment questions for this developmental stage include:

- What type of activities are satisfying for the couple?
- In what type of social and family activities does the couple engage?
- Does the couple look back on their lives with satisfaction and feelings of accomplishment?
- How does the couple adjust to loss?

Some wellness diagnoses for this developmental stage are

~ *Progressive participation in satisfying service activities*
~ *Maintenance of intergenerational relationships*

~ *Satisfaction with family life as lived*
~ *Progressive adaptation to changes in family lifestyle occurring from loss*

CASE STUDY

This case study is presented to demonstrate the use of wellness nursing diagnoses with the normal family. However, for the sake of brevity, all aspects of family life will not be included.

Janet and Howard Green live in a modest three-bedroom brick home with their son Jimmy who is 3 years old. Janet, 28 years old, is in the 36th week of a normal pregnancy, and from the ultrasound results, the family expects a girl. Currently, Janet is on maternity leave from her secretarial position. Howard, 32 years old, works at the local soft-drink bottling factory where he has just been promoted to shipping supervisor on the evening shift.

Janet and Howard have a number of friends who are their age and are beginning families. Therefore, when Janet meets with her friends, discussions often center around availability of child care facilities and baby-sitters, ways to discipline small children, and pre-natal classes, as well as routine daily living such as cooking, sewing, and leisure activities.

On the other hand, Howard and his friends discuss sports, work, and hobbies; but they are also becoming more aware of the difficulties of finding time to be with their children, especially if they work evening shifts. They want to be involved in their wives' pregnancies and often show each other the ultra-sound pictures they have received at prenatal visits.

Janet and Howard have been married for 5 years and have developed a pattern of communication that allows them to share their joys, concerns, and common goals. They enjoy being together and plan time each weekend for family activities. Although their own parents live several hours away, they frequently talk to them by phone.

Before Jimmy was born, they discussed ways they would share his care, so that he would learn from both his parents. They are satisfied with the way they have parented Jimmy and plan to continue the same pattern, although they know the addition of a new child will make it necessary to make some changes.

Janet and Howard have mutually created a plan that will enable Howard to be present during labor and delivery. He has arranged for a fellow worker to take over for him if Janet goes into labor while he is at work. The hospital has provided him with a beeper so he will know when Janet is ready to go to the hospital.

Both Janet and Howard want Jimmy to be incorporated into the new baby's care, but they are somewhat concerned about sibling rivalry. The local hospital has sibling classes and Jimmy is registered to attend them in the next week. Jimmy has felt the baby move, has been encouraged to talk to the fetus, and has helped in planning the nursery. Janet has bought a new toy for Jimmy that she will give him when the baby is brought home.

Janet's physician recommends that the husband and wife spend one evening alone before Janet comes back for her 6-week postpartum checkup. Both Janet and Howard recognize that they need to find time to be alone without their children and have discussed ways that this can be accomplished. They both remember that when Jimmy was born, they felt they neglected each other at times. Fortunately, they were able to discuss these feelings and to resolve the potential conflict. Based on past experience, they are trying to find ways to avoid a similar situation.

Janet and Howard recognize the need for a balance of time alone for each partner, time for the partners to be together without the children, time for Jimmy to be with his parents without the new baby, and family time for the entire family unit. They wonder where all this time will come from, particularly when Janet goes back to work. However, they continue to plan and talk about their feelings, realizing that nothing will be perfect, but recognizing that planning may make the transition easier from a group of three to a group of four.

When assessing this family unit, several wellness diagnoses arise: *adjusting to changes in family config-*

uration, progressive development of family child care patterns, and *progressive inclusion of child in family discussions and decisions.* Goals for this family could be (a) continued adjustment to changes in family configuration, (b) continued development of family child care patterns, and (c) continued inclusion of child in family discussions and decisions. Nursing interventions would include exploration of ways to adjust to changes in family configuration, information on a variety of child care patterns, and praise for inclusion of the child in family decisions.

SUMMARY

This chapter has focused on wellness diagnoses for families. Two methods of family assessment have been presented. A number of wellness diagnoses have been proposed using the developmental stages of the family. Examples of the relationship among wellness diagnoses, behaviors, and interventions for families are presented in Table 15.1 (see overleaf).

References

Bomar, P.J. (1990). Perspectives on family health promotion. *Family and Community Health, 12*(4), 1–11.

Caudle, P., and Grover, S. (1992). Care of the family client. In M.J. Clark (ed.), *Nursing in the Community* (pp. 393–418). Norwalk, CT: Appleton & Lange.

Curran, D. (1983). *Traits of a Healthy Family.* Minneapolis: Winston Press.

Curran, D. (1985). *Stress and the Health Family.* Minneapolis: Winston Press.

Duvall, E.M. (1977). *Marriage and Family Development,* 5th ed. Philadelphia: Lippincott.

Duvall, E.M., and Miller, B.C. (1985). *Marriage and Family Development,* 6th ed. New York: Harper & Row.

Friedman, M.M., and Miller, K. (1992). Family development theory. In M.M. Friedman (ed.), *Family Nursing: Theory and Practice,* 3rd ed. (pp. 81–111). Norwalk, CT: Appleton & Lange.

Gordon, M. (1994). *Nursing Diagnosis: Process and Application*. St. Louis: Mosby-Yearbook.

Lynch, I., and Tiedje, L.B. (1991). Working with multiproblem families: An intervention model for community health nurses. *Public Health Nursing, 8*, 147–153.

McCubbin, M.A. (1993). Family stress theory and the development of nursing knowledge about family adaptation. In S.L. Feetham, S.B. Meister, J.M. Bell, and C.L. Gilliss (eds.), *The Nursing of Families* (pp. 354–364). Newbury Park, CA: Sage.

Nettle, C., Pavelich, J., Jones, N., and Beltz, C. (1993). Family as client: Using Gordon's health pattern typology. *Journal of Community Health Nursing, 10*(1), 53–61.

Neuman, B. (1995). *The Neuman Systems Model*, 3rd ed. Norwalk, CT: Appleton & Lange.

Nursing Diagnoses: Definitions and Classification 1995–1996 (1994). Philadelphia: North American Nursing Diagnosis Association.

Petze, C.F. (1984). Health promotion for the well family. *Nursing Clinics of North America, 19*(2), 229–237.

Ross, B., and Cobb, K.L. (1990). *Family Nursing: A Nursing Process Approach*. Redwood City, CA: Addison-Wesley.

Smilkstein, G. (1984). The physician and family function assessment. *Family Systems Medicine, 2*, 236–278.

Stanhope, M., and Lancaster, J. (1992). *Community Health Nursing: Process and Practice for Promoting Health*, 3rd ed. St. Louis: Mosby-Yearbook.

Thomas, R.B., Barnard, K.E., and Sumner, G.A. (1993). Family nursing diagnosis as a framework for family assessment. In S.L. Featham, S.B. Meister, J.M. Bell, and C.L. Gilliss (eds.), *The Nursing of Families* (pp. 127–136). Newbury Park, CA: Sage.

Table 15.1. Relationships Among Selected Wellness Nursing Diagnoses, Behaviors, and Interventions: Families

Wellness Nursing Diagnosis	Family Behaviors	Nursing Interventions
Progressive development of mutually satisfying relationship	Couple has a pattern of open communication where perceptions, thoughts, and feelings can be shared without fear of reprisal	Praise couple for open communication
	Couple engages in conflict resolution that respects each member of the dyad	Discuss methods of conflict resolution
		Help couple identify individual needs as well as mutual needs
	Couple begins to develop patterns of living that allow for individual as well as mutual needs	Discuss ways that individual and mutual needs can be met without conflict
Beginning development of the family unit	Couple spends time together developing mutual interests	Encourage identification/development of mutual goals and interests
	Couple relies on themselves for decision making without extended family input	Reinforce self-reliance as a couple rather than reliance on parents
	Couple identifies goals they wish to accomplish	When appropriate, guide couple in decision making
		Assist with goal development as needed

Developing ties to extended family	Couple incorporates extended family into some of their activities	Encourage developing ties to extended family while helping the couple to maintain their separate identity
	Couple recognizes needs of extended family members and helps to meet those needs	Help couple identify those things they can do alone and those things where they need help
	Couple is able to accept help from extended family as needed	
Increasing allocation by couple of time alone without the infant	Couple sets time aside without infant to meet intimacy needs	Encourage couple to find ways to spend time as a couple
	Couple shares feelings with each other about being new parents and how they can combine roles of parent and lover	Explore ways that time can be allocated to meet needs of the couple
		Discuss role changes with the couple and encourage sharing of feelings about those roles
Progressive development of family child care patterns	Couple discusses beliefs about parenting roles	Encourage discussion of beliefs about child care
	Couple respects each other's beliefs about child care and identifies patterns of child care they can accept	Share types of child care patterns

(continued)

263

Wellness Nursing Diagnosis	Family Behaviors	Nursing Interventions
Progressive development of family child care patterns (cont'd.)	Couple decides how child care will be divided between the two parents	Discuss differences between ways men and women handle infants and reassure couple that both ways contribute to a child's development
		Help couple reach decisions about division of labor
Increasing social interaction appropriate for children's ages and abilities	As a group, family participates in activities outside the home	Encourage group participation in family activities
	Family provides opportunities for children to interact with other children	Discuss need for diverse activities to enhance child development
		Explore opportunities for interaction with other children
Progressive inclusion of children in family discussions and decisions	Family allows children to express individual needs	Discuss age-appropriate ways that children can be involved in family decisions
	As children grow, they are encouraged to provide input into family decision making	Praise inclusion of children in conversations
	Children participate in family discussion at	

264

mealtime

	Children are prepared for the new baby	Explore with family changes that will occur as family size or configuration changes
	Family provides time for each child to be recognized and feel important	Suggest alternative ways that needs of individual children can be met either separately or within the family group
	Time is allocated for each child to have some time alone with either or both parents	
	Older children are helped to include younger children in activities without exclusion of their own particular needs	
Adapting individual roles within the family to accommodate changes in family configuration or size	Family roles are discussed as family size or configuration changes	
Increasing utilization of family and community resources	Family finds ways to conserve time, resources, and money in order to meet needs of increasing family size	Suggest ways to conserve resources or to expand resources through sharing with other families, or bartering time and resources
	Family is aware of community resources and knows how to use them as necessary	Discuss community resources with family to help them know what is available and how to use them

(continued)

265

Wellness Nursing Diagnosis	Family Behaviors	Nursing Interventions
Increasing ability of individual family members to give and take in order to meet each other's needs	Family members can communicate their own needs	With family unit, discuss individual and group needs
	Family members can describe each other's needs	Help family members define their responsibilities toward other family members
	Family members can compromise in order to meet each other's needs	Suggest ways that both individual and group needs can be met
Maintaining balance between independent and dependent needs of children	Family recognizes that children have desire to be independent yet often maintain dependency needs	Discuss developmental tasks of children and adolescents
	Family encourages children to develop age-appropriate independence	Explore behaviors that indicate increasing need for independence
	Family continues to meet children's dependency needs as appropriate	Suggest ways to expand opportunities for independence that provide safety and security for children
Continued commitment to family values	Family as a unit clarifies family values as necessary	Facilitate discussion of family values
	Parents help children clarify personal values	Praise family for making value statements
		Suggest ways that family values can be

		strengthened or reinforced
	Consistencies and inconsistencies between family members' behavior and family values are discussed.	Assist family members in identifying inconsistencies between behaviors and values
Integration of new family member	Children's spouses are welcomed into family unit	Reinforce inclusion of children's spouses in extended family
	Children's spouses are included in family discussions and in mutual decision making as appropriate	Encourage family members to get to know children's spouses through sharing of common goals and interests
Beginning reestablishment of a mutually satisfying couple relationship	Couple refocuses on dyadic relationship by spending time together	Encourage couple to spend time together now that children are gone from home
	Couple shares current interests and goals	Reinforce mutual goal development
	Couple reaffirms their commitment to each other	Praise continued commitment
Progressive reestablishment of a mutually satisfying couple relationship	Couple balances individual needs with needs for the couple	Reinforce need for balance
		Explore ways that couple can continue to meet these needs

(continued)

Wellness Nursing Diagnosis	Family Behaviors	Nursing Interventions
Progressive reestablishment of a mutually satisfying couple relationship (cont'd.)	Couple provides emotional support for each other	Reinforce couple's commitment to each other
Progressive participation in satisfying service activities	Couple identifies service activities in which they can be involved	Encourage couple to find satisfying activities within physical limitations
	Couple expresses satisfaction with service activities	Provide list of service activities if needed
		Share couple's satisfaction with their achievements
Maintenance of intergenerational relationships	Family member(s) maintains ties with younger generation(s)	Encourage generations to communicate with each other
	Family member(s) contributes to younger generation's knowledge as appropriate	Help generations identify what each can contribute to the other
	Family member(s) receives help from younger generation(s) as appropriate	
Satisfaction with family life as lived	Family member(s) reminisces about family activities	Encourage reminiscence
		Reinforce satisfaction with accomplishments

Progressive adaption to changes in family lifestyle occurring from loss

Family member(s) describes satisfaction with family life

Family member(s) is proud of family accomplishments

Family member(s) identifies losses and seeks to resolve loss

Family member(s) makes appropriate changes in lifestyle to accommodate loss

Praise family for accomplishments

Listen to family member(s) describe loss and how it impacts lifestyle

Suggest alternative ways to adapt lifestyle to accommodate loss

269

Karen M. Stolte: WELLNESS NURSING
DIAGNOSIS FOR HEALTH PROMOTION.
© 1996 Lippincott–Raven Publishers.

16
~

Wellness Nursing Diagnoses for Communities

Community health nurses have as one of their concerns the health of the community. Moving from an individual focus to a group focus to a community focus involves higher and higher levels of complexity. Working with the community as the unit of service means attention is directed at the systems level. Change must occur in the community rather than at the individual or group level.

Although attempts have been made to define community and to look at nursing diagnoses in the community, much of this work is in its infancy. Nevertheless, the reader can find information in community health textbooks. There are also books written on the community-as-client. The complete assessment of communities is beyond the scope of this book. The reader is referred to the undergraduate community health textbooks that discuss assessment. Because of the limited amount of information on community wellness diagnoses, literature from the past as well as present is included.

~ Definition of the Community

Cassells (1993) notes that the community has three dimensions: a group of people, a location in space and time, and a social system. This group of people shares common characteristics that result in collective goals and activities.

A community has a defined physical or geographical location. Various kinds of boundaries define the parameters of the community. The boundaries and composition of the people who live in a community may change over time. Therefore, time is considered in the definition of the community.

As a social system, a community is composed of many interrelated subsystems, which in turn carry out the functions of the community. Socialization, goal attainment, and social support are often accomplished through these subsystems.

~ *Community Competence*

Since the focus of this book is on wellness, definitions of community competence will be presented as a way of assessing community strengths. A healthy community is better able to promote the growth and development of groups and individuals than is an unhealthy one (Stanhope and Lancaster, 1992). A competent community is one in which its interdependent parts can:

1. Collaborate in community problem identification
2. Achieve consensus on goals and priorities
3. Agree on ways to reach the goals
4. Collaborate in carrying out the actions (Cottrell, 1976, p. 197)

Cottrell goes on to say that there are eight essential conditions that must exist to some degree in a community for it to function effectively:

1. COMMITMENT — Individuals can see that the community has an impact on their lives and that whatever affects it will affect them; they have a significant role in the community; and they see positive results from their community efforts.
2. SELF-OTHER AWARENESS — Each community component knows its identity and how it relates to the other components of the community.

3. ARTICULATENESS — Each component of the community can articulate its attitudes and intentions as well as state how it relates to other components of the community.

4. COMMUNICATION — Components of the community can not only send messages, but they can put themselves in the other's place in order to see how their message will be received.

5. CONFLICT CONTAINMENT AND ACCOMMODATION — When conflict exists, it is "kept in bounds" and efforts at resolution continue.

6. PARTICIPATION — As components of the community interact, they become committed, define goals, and find ways to reach those goals.

7. MANAGEMENT OF RELATIONS WITH THE LARGER SOCIETY— Any community is a part of a larger social system and must determine how it fits within that system. It utilizes the input from the larger system while acting to reduce threats from that system.

8. MACHINERY FOR FACILITATING PARTICIPANT INTERACTION AND DECISION MAKING — Constant monitoring assures that mechanisms exist to ensure communication and interaction among the various components of the community.

In like manner, Spradley (1985) maintains that conditions for a healthy community include awareness of community identity, problem-solving ability, recognition of subgroups and their value, open communication channels, conflict resolution skills, participation by all citizens, and promotion of high-level wellness.

~ Community Wellness Nursing Diagnoses in the Literature

Although authors often present methods of community assessment and community nursing diagnoses, few include wellness diagnoses. One notable exception is Neufeld and Harrison

(1990), who consider both problem-oriented and wellness-oriented diagnoses in their discussion of nursing diagnoses for aggregates and groups. Their wellness diagnoses are *"high school students have a potential for successfully achieving developmental task (ability to parent),"* *"women working in XXXX have a potential for achieving optimum physical fitness,"* and *"participants in XXX club in the XX Seniors apartment have optimum nutritional status"* (p. 252). These diagnoses pertain to subsystems within the community. Using a host–environment framework, they list a number of contributing factors from both the host and the environment for each diagnosis.

Porter (1987) asserts that community diagnoses include two steps: (1) to determine the health status of the population group and (2) to determine how well matched are the population's needs and existing services. In keeping with this format, Clark (1992) incorporates use of wellness diagnoses in looking at the health status of a community or target group. Using assessment data indicating that immunization services are available in the community and the population has a high immunization level, she arrives at the following diagnosis: *"need–service match due to accessibility and use of immunization services"* (p. 434).

NANDA (1994) has one community nursing diagnosis that is somewhat related to community strengths but still is based on at least one deficit in the community. This diagnosis is *potential for enhanced community coping* (NANDA, p. 55).

∼ Assessment of Community Strengths

In the following paragraphs, several methods of community assessment are mentioned. Two wellness diagnoses related to community process solving are given for the reader to consider. As with the other chapters in this book, only the response portion of the diagnosis is included. The condition portion will vary with the particular situation.

The use of nursing models for assessment of the community is limited because most models were designed for individual clients. However, Hanchett (1990) reviews the use of four nursing models using the community as the client. Neuman's (1995) system model is cited more frequently than the other models when assessing the community.

In general, nurses do not work alone in the community, but are part of a larger interdisciplinary team. Interventions are directed at global economic, social, political, and educational levels. Nurses collaborate with interested parties in program planning, influencing policy, and identifying available or needed resources. The goal is delivery of services as determined by aggregates or community use of an epidemiological approach of cost/benefit ratio prediction. Examples of targets for interventions may be school systems, occupational groups, industrial sites, or churches.

To arrive at community nursing diagnoses, emphasis must be on the collective health of the community rather than health of individuals. The health of an individual is considered in light of how it will affect the entire community. Therefore, there are major differences in assessment of the community compared to assessment of an individual. Data about the community come from many sources, ranging from census data and phone books to community self-studies and surveys.

A variety of methods are used for community assessment. Most community health textbooks include at least one method. Cassells (1993, pp. 86–87) suggests the following categories for community assessment:

GEOGRAPHY — terrain and climate
POPULATION — demographic characteristics, size
ENVIRONMENT — water, air quality, housing, waste disposal
INDUSTRY — type, employment levels
EDUCATION — literacy rates, kinds of schools, special education services
RECREATION — parks, playgrounds, special facilities
RELIGION — churches and synagogues, community programs
COMMUNICATION — newspapers, radio and television stations

TRANSPORTATION — bus lines, emergency services, handicapped services

PUBLIC SERVICES — fire, police, utilities

POLITICAL ORGANIZATIONS — structure, voting procedures

COMMUNITY DEVELOPMENT OR PLANNING — activities

DISASTER PROGRAMS — American Red Cross, disaster plans

HEALTH STATISTICS — births, mortality and morbidity

SOCIAL PROBLEMS — crime, drugs, gangs

HEALTH MANPOWER — who and where

HEALTH PROFESSIONAL ORGANIZATIONS — composition and type

COMMUNITY SERVICES — inpatient and outpatient services, preventive programs

Spradley (1985) proposes dividing the community into various systems and then assessing these systems: health system, family system, economic system, educational system, religious system, welfare system, political system, recreation system, legal system, and communication system. In many respects, this format is similar to that of Cassells. Other authors use Gordon's (1994) functional health patterns for community assessment.

Cassells' format provides the content areas to be assessed in a community. Assessment questions related to community problem solving might include:

- Who are the leaders in the community? Formal? Informal?
- What kind of groups exist in the community to address community problems, define goals, and initiate action?
- What is the composition of these groups: consumers, professionals, industry representatives, etc.?
- What kind of action is taken by these groups?

Wellness diagnoses related to community process could be

~ *Progressive community interaction for problem solving and goal identification*

~ *Progressive participation in community goal-directed activities*

The assessment data provide the information about specific goals, particular problems, and actual activities. If the nurse wants more specificity in the diagnosis, the goals and activities can be included.

Looking at specific groups rather than the total community is probably more workable as long as group actions are related back to the community goal. Evaluation is done in terms of changes in the total community. The following case study will examine specific groups rather than a total community.

CASE STUDY

Waterton is a community of approximately 250,000 people. Although the population is mostly Caucasian, there are small pockets of ethnic groups including Afro-Americans and Hispanics. Many young families live in the community and have limited incomes because the majority of jobs are in blue-collar industry.

From examining city–county health department statistics, community leaders have become aware of increases in high-risk pregnancies. Infant morbidity and mortality statistics have also risen in the past 2 years. There is a recognized lack of prenatal care since the majority of women seek care after the 20th week of pregnancy or have no prenatal care. In addition, there is a high rate of adolescent pregnancy.

The city officials arranged multidisciplinary meetings of professionals from the three local hospitals, community health nurses who direct a prenatal clinic at the city–county health department, legislative groups, school officials, and interested citizens to discuss the problem and propose possible solutions. As a result of these meetings, the need to improve maternity services for adolescents was established.

In order to address this need, subgroups were formed. These subgroups came from legislative groups, school systems, church groups, community health agencies such as freestanding and hospital clinics, and agencies responsible for transportation. Health professionals from a variety of disciplines such as nursing, medicine, public health, and dietetics; adolescent consumers of maternity care; clergy; teachers; and administrative leaders from the community, health agencies, and transportation services worked together in these groups, so that all points of view could be considered. The plans from each subgroup were sent to community planning groups to verify that coordination of activities was done, duplication of efforts was reduced, and each subgroup had the resources to accomplish its task.

As a result of all these activities, the community was able to increase the number of sites where prenatal care could be obtained, improve the access to transportation to these prenatal sites, increase the number of hours (including evenings and weekends) that prenatal care could be obtained, provide programs in the school systems that focused on the need for prenatal care, provide counseling services for pregnant adolescents in the school systems or with local church groups, and make legislative changes that helped finance prenatal care for those unable to afford it. Suggested wellness diagnoses for this community are *progressive improvement of access to prenatal services, increasing communication between professional and consumer groups, increasing subgroup conflict resolution ability,* and *increasing pride in community action.*

Upon evaluation, some of the indicators that the goal of improved maternity services with improved maternity outcomes was reached were reduction in mortality/morbidity statistics, fewer high-risk pregnancies, and a higher incidence of pregnant adolescents receiving prenatal care before the 20th week of pregnancy.

SUMMARY

This chapter has focused on wellness diagnoses for the community. A description of the competent community is provided. Examples of the relationship among wellness diagnoses, behaviors, and interventions for a community are presented in Table 16.1.

References

Cassells, H.B. (1993). Nursing process in the community. In J.M. Swanson and M. Albrecht (eds.), *Community Health Nursing: Promoting the Health of Aggregates* (pp. 81–108). Philadelphia: Saunders.

Clark, M.J. (1992). *Nursing in the Community*. Norwalk, CT: Appleton & Lange.

Cottrell, L.S. (1976). The competent community. In B.H. Kaplan, R.N. Wilson, and A.H. Leighton (eds.), *Further Explorations in Social Psychiatry* (pp. 195–209). New York: Basic Books. **[AU: My page number correction okay?]**

Gordon, M. (1994). *Nursing Diagnosis: Process and Application*. St. Louis: Mosby-Yearbook.

Hanchett, E.S. (1990). Nursing models and community as client. *Nursing Science Quarterly, 3*(2), 67–72.

Neufeld, A., and Harrison, M.J. (1990). The development of nursing diagnoses for aggregates and groups. *Public Health Nursing, 7*(4), 251–255.

Neuman, B. (1995). *The Neuman Systems Model*, 3rd ed. Norwalk, CT: Appleton & Lange.

Nursing Diagnoses: Definitions and Classification 1995–1996 (1994). Philadelphia: North American Nursing Diagnosis Association.

Porter, E.J. (1987). Administrative diagnosis—Implications for the public's health. *Public Health Nursing, 4*(4), 247–256.

Spradley, B.W. (1985). *Community Health Nursing*, 2nd ed. Boston: Little, Brown & Co.

Stanhope, M., and Lancaster, J. (1992). *Community Health Nursing: Process and Practice for Promoting Health*, 3rd ed. St. Louis: Mosby-Yearbook.

Table 16.1. Relationships Among Selected Wellness Nursing Diagnoses, Behaviors, and Interventions: Community

Wellness Nursing Diagnosis	Community Behaviors	Nursing Interventions
Progressive community interaction for problem solving and goal identification	Multidisciplinary groups are formed to identify community problems	Suggest composition of groups
		Work with other professionals to facilitate group decision making and goal development
	Multidisciplinary groups define community goals	
		Suggest ways groups can work together to plan community action
	Multidisciplinary groups work together to plan for goal achievement	
		Suggest alternative plans for goal achievement
Progressive participation in community goal-directed activities	Multidisciplinary groups are formed that have authority to take action toward goal achievement	Suggest composition of groups
		Coordinate activities to ensure maximum participation of group members
	Groups formulate and execute a plan of action	
		Facilitate group process to achieve mutual goal setting
	Groups report activities to community leaders	
		Coordinate group activities to maximize efforts toward goal achievement

279

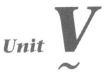

*W*ellness Nursing Diagnosis in Literature
~

17
~

Review and Critique of Wellness Nursing Diagnosis Literature

The following literature review will focus on the small, but growing, group of articles related specifically to wellness nursing diagnoses. The purpose of this review is to familiarize the reader with the available literature, demonstrate the variety of approaches used for writing wellness nursing diagnoses, and discuss various problems and limitations with these suggested ways to write wellness diagnoses.

Since writing wellness diagnoses is in its infancy, no one framework has been accepted. Some proposed frameworks include using the problem, etiology, sign/symptoms format proposed by Gordon (1994); including criteria in the wellness diagnosis by adding the words *as evidenced by;* changing qualifiers such as ineffective, inadequate, or unhealthy in currently accepted NANDA problem-oriented nursing diagnoses to positive qualifiers such as effective, adequate, or healthy; or using a modified Mundinger and Jauron (1975) framework, substituting a healthy response for the unhealthy one suggested by the authors.

In the articles cited, some authors describe how to write wellness nursing diagnoses, others give examples, and still others discuss the possibility of including healthy states when writing nursing diagnoses but give no examples. The articles are grouped according to approach to wellness nursing diagnoses or methods of writing these diagnoses.

~ Advocacy of Wellness Nursing Diagnoses

The first articles to be discussed include those whose authors advocate the use of wellness nursing diagnoses, or at least recognize the possibility that healthy client responses are within the domain of nursing. Sometimes examples of wellness diagnoses are given; sometimes they are not.

Using the concept of unitary person, Guzzetta, Bunton, Prinkey, Sherer, and Seifert (1988) describe nine response patterns for the human being. They consider the human as an open system in mutual interaction with the environment. The nine response patterns allow for both wellness and illness behaviors. No nursing diagnoses are included in the article.

Bestard and Courtenay (1990) define wellness diagnoses as statements about client strengths that are derived from healthy behaviors. They believe that nursing goals are directed toward maintaining or enhancing the client's level of functioning. An example of a wellness nursing diagnosis is *"positive self-esteem related to continued independence and healthy relationships with family"* (p. 25).

Popkess-Vawter and Pinnell (1987) define nursing diagnosis as a conclusion that describes "human responses to actual or potential health concerns and practices" (p. 1216). They envision health concerns as a continuum including problems and strengths. In addition, they believe wellness nursing diagnoses can provide a way to measure wellness services. Taking a similar stance, Taylor-Loughran (1990) concludes that a nursing diagnosis is "a component of the nursing process which is concerned with a wide range of health-related responses in sick and well persons" (p. 71). She states that the element of judgment provided in the nursing diagnosis allows for consideration of healthy responses, not just problems.

Lee and Frenn (1987) also maintain that patterns of human responses are both positive and negative. They point out that nursing diagnoses are needed that reflect both patterns. Recognizing that nursing diagnoses help define and organize knowledge, they use the term *positive nursing diagnosis* to incorporate health promotion and wellness activities in community health nursing. Examples of wellness diagnoses cited in the article include *"readiness for growth"* and *"positive self-care strategies"* (p. 985).

Roy and Andrews (1991) suggest that nursing diagnoses may be used for both effective and ineffective responses when using the Roy model of nursing. The example of a positive nursing diagnosis given is *"effective coping strategies to grieve the loss of a limb"* (p. 40).

Stolte (1986a) advocates a dual approach to nursing diagnosis that allows for both wellness-oriented and problem-oriented diagnoses for each client. Such an approach permits the nurse to identify client strengths as well as weaknesses. For writing wellness nursing diagnoses, she suggests the Mundinger and Jauron (1975) nursing diagnosis format that includes a response to a condition but substitutes a healthy response for an unhealthy one. Using the term *positive diagnosis*, she cites examples from each clinical area such as *"successful, rapid convalescence related to philosophy of positive thinking"* (adult health nursing); *"joy related to birth of a healthy baby"* (maternity nursing); *"integrity related to satisfaction of having raised a family well, having planned for retirement, and being content with decisions made during life"* (*community health nursing*); *"imitation of feminine role models and sexual curiosity related to establishing feminine identity"* (*pediatric nursing*); *and* *"developing self-awareness related to trust and respect among group members"* (*psychiatric–mental health nursing*) (*p. 27*).

In a later article, Popkess-Vawter (1991) again emphasizes the need for wellness nursing diagnoses. She suggests the health-illness-wellness model proposed by Hornberger (1989) as a framework to demonstrate how wellness nursing diagnoses can be used in all clinical areas across the scope of nursing. This model assumes that all persons have some degree of wellness. Popkess notes that in situations where clients demonstrate wellness behaviors, these behaviors may not be firmly established nor may supports be present to help sustain these behaviors. In both instances, nursing care is needed to reinforce wellness patterns. Wellness nursing diagnoses provide the guidance for such nursing care. A number of wellness nursing diagnoses are presented such as *"adequate individual coping related to church activities and regular visits from new church friends"* (p. 23), and increased *"activity tolerance related to gaining weight associated with improved sucking reflex"* (p. 24).

~ Wellnesss Diagnosis Framework of Healthy and Unhealthy Responses

Several authors suggest modification of adjectives for client responses in nursing diagnoses to allow for either a positive or a negative response. Even though Popkess-Vawter (1981, 1984) writes about assessment of client strengths for the purpose of providing holistic care, she uses many of the diagnoses types that were originally written for problem situations. She affirms the use of adjectives such as effective, appropriate, or adequate to describe the client strength. Examples given in the 1984 article include: *"airway clearance, effective"*; *"gas exchange, adequate"*; and *"sleep pattern, healthy"* (p. 438). Unfortunately, the adjectives described may be subjective, rather than objective, conclusions because one nurse may describe behavior as effective or healthy and another nurse may not. Most importantly, the terms *effective*, *adequate*, and *healthy* are nonspecific terms that give little direction for continued care. Nevertheless, Popkess-Vawter was one of the first writers to advocate wellness nursing diagnoses and she believes the nurse can help the client rehabilitate or adjust to current health problems by building on his or her strengths.

Lyons and Hester (1987) provide a list of nursing diagnoses that include both healthy and unhealthy responses, and the response chosen depends on client data. Some examples include *"sound (reduced) nutritional status related to quality of foods eaten"*; *"good (impaired) physical health related to functional integrity of body"*; *"beneficial (inadequate) sleep time related to quantity of sleep"* (pp. 152–153). When describing the need for positive diagnoses, they assert that a nursing diagnosis is concerned with the client's health status and, as such, this definition allows for diagnosis of a positive state as well as for a deficit state of health. They also declare that if a positive state is included, nursing diagnoses work well in primary care settings and can be used to increase nursing accountability.

In a Delphi survey of consensus on wellness and health promotion nursing diagnoses, Frenn, Jacobs, Lee, Sanger, and Strong (1987) found that controversy exists among nurses identified as experts in health promotion about whether or not wellness diagnoses should be used. Those respondents who supported the use of wellness diagnoses stated that these diagnoses (1) provide an opportunity for nurses to give reinforcement and support, (2) are needed for healthy populations, (3) show that nursing has a place in health promotion, and (4) encourage nursing interventions that help the client maintain a wellness state. Those nurses who did not support the use of wellness nursing diagnoses believed that if the client were healthy, a nurse was not needed. Nevertheless, nurses who work in health promotion and wellness settings were capable of formulating such diagnoses. Seventy-six possible wellness nursing diagnoses are listed in the article. In these diagnoses, a combination of healthy and unhealthy responses was used, culminating in conclusions about whether behavior is effective or ineffective. Some examples are *"sleep/rest pattern, effective/ineffective"*; and *"stress management, effective/ineffective"* (p. 157). In contrast, some diagnoses in the article only describe healthy responses such as *"grieving, functional"*; *"nutritional patterns, adequate"*; and *"anticipatory role transition (specify), desire for future growth"*

(p. 157). Use of vague terms such as effective or adequate may result in miscommunication since a common definition of those terms probably does not exist. In addition, an ambiguous nursing diagnosis leads to vague goals, which makes it difficult to determine, at a later date, if the goals for care are met.

~ Describing Specific Health Behaviors in a Wellness Diagnosis

Some authors propose wellness nursing diagnoses that describe, in detail, specific health behaviors of the client. Gleit and Tatro (1981) define a nursing diagnosis as a "statement of an individual's response that is healthy or actually or potentially unhealthy and which independent nursing interventions can help to reinforce or strengthen in the direction of optimal health" (p. 456). Amplifying the definition to include both healthy and unhealthy responses provides the nurse with an opportunity to assess patient strengths and to reinforce these strengths when planning care. The nursing diagnosis given is *"progressive relaxation for ten minutes upon arising and two hours after dinner related to stress management and psychological well-being"* (p. 456). The response portion of this diagnosis describes a particular stress management behavior that leaves little room for change. Therefore, one would question why a nurse is needed. In addition, the diagnosis seems rather long. Conceptually, description of specific behaviors seems more appropriate for goals than for diagnoses. Perhaps a more useful diagnosis would be *practicing stress management behaviors related to wellness beliefs* because it allows flexibility in type of stress management behaviors used by the client and is at the level of abstraction typically seen in nursing diagnoses.

In a second article, Tatro and Gleit (1983) again incorporate specific health behaviors into their style of diagnosis. Examples of such diagnoses include *"riding a bicycle for one hour each day related to knowledge of aerobic fitness benefits"* and *"engaging in daily meditation related to a feeling of self-control and* composure" (p. 8). As in the first article, these diagnoses seem extremely long and unwieldy and delineate specific behaviors rather than focusing on responses that reflect clusters of behaviors.

Flagler and Nicoll (1990) present both positive and negative nursing diagnoses related to maternal identity formation. However, these diagnoses are very long because they include the behaviors that describe the response. One also wonders for what purpose the positive diagnoses are designed since there is no evidence that a nurse is needed. The diagnoses are purely descriptive and do not provide a foundation for planning and intervention. An example of a positive diagnosis is *"positive alteration in body image self evidenced by wearing appropriate clothing and shoes to accommodate changing body"* (p. 274).

Martens (1986) also promotes a system of writing nursing diagnoses that describes, in detail, the behaviors that provide evidence for the nursing diagnosis. She asserts that individuals have more strengths than problems and behaviors that maintain wellness need to be reinforced. In order to promote complete understanding of the client, she proposes presentation of a balance of nursing diagnoses reflecting both weaknesses and strengths. Examples of diagnostic statements that reflect strengths include *"desire to maintain independence evidenced by high involvement in decision making and active search for information about illness and therapy"* and *"active support system including family and peer involvement with client evidenced by daily visits and participation in problem solving"* (p. 193). Unfortunately, these diagnoses tend to be lengthy. If a diagnosis is too long, its purpose as a concise statement of assessment data is lost. Nevertheless, the basic idea of inclusion of a balance of strengths and weaknesses in the nursing diagnosis list is appealing. Martens also describes diagnoses that emphasize the client's potential for healthy behaviors. Such diagnoses include *"effective coping with aging process, potential for growth"*; *"adequate nutrition, potential for improvement"*; *"effective stress reduction, potential for better management"* (p. 193).

Keeling (1988) is one of a few authors who describes wellness diagnoses for acute care settings. Her diagnoses are similar to Martens (1986) in that she provides descriptions of client behaviors and environmental variables such as *"potential for compliance with low-cholesterol, low-sodium diet related to wife's concern for her own hypertension and her stated desire to change the family's dietary habits"* (p. 32).

Using a different nursing diagnosis format, Stolte (1989) describes use of wellness nursing diagnoses in situations where the client is quite ill. Two examples are given: *"progression of healing myocardium related to ability to manage myocardial oxygen supply and demand"* and *"progressive weaning from ventilator related to willingness to participate in weaning plan"* (pp. 79–80).

~ Clinical Areas and Wellness Diagnoses

One of the reasons for an increasing interest in wellness nursing diagnoses is the lack of ability to use problem-oriented diagnoses in settings where the clients are generally healthy or in areas where the focus is on health promotion. In those instances, nurses often avoid the use of nursing diagnoses since the NANDA taxonomy does not meet their needs. Allen (1989) reports ways that community health nurses have modified existing diagnoses or developed new ones to incorporate the concepts of promotion, prevention, and protection. Some changes include modification of existing NANDA diagnoses to include positive modifiers such as adequate or healthy, addition of defining characteristics pertinent to health, or use of taxonomies developed by sources other than NANDA. A wellness diagnosis used by one group of nurses is *"knowledge or ability to use information regarding (specify)"* (p. 41). The specifics in the diagnosis relate to functional health patterns assessed by the nurse prior to making the diagnosis. This diagnosis is included in a category of diagnoses about the healthy individual/family.

When discussing aggregate nursing diagnoses for community health, Ridenour (1994) noted that refinement and development of a wellness focus is relevant because it encourages client involvement and dialogue between client and provider. In like fashion, Neufeld and Harrison (1994) believe there is a need to develop a taxonomy of wellness diagnoses that can be used with groups and individuals in community health settings. Although they found that nurses working in community-based programs listed both wellness and deficit diagnoses when given a questionnaire about nursing diagnoses, the wellness diagnoses were difficult to measure or described deficits that needed to be corrected rather than focusing on wellness per se.

Articles exist in the maternity nursing literature related to the use of wellness nursing diagnoses with these healthy clients. Zetelmaier (1983) mentions the difficulty that maternity nurses have in using the NANDA-approved list of nursing diagnoses because it focuses primarily on problems and potential problems. Nicoletti (1991) and Stolte (1986b) reaffirm this difficulty. Since Standard II in the American Nurses Association's *Standards of Clinical Nursing Practice* (1991) includes nursing diagnoses, such diagnoses need to be used in all clinical areas in order to demonstrate quality care.

To alleviate the problem of lack of use of nursing diagnoses in maternity nursing, Stolte (1986b) advocates use of wellness nursing diagnoses for these clients. Two examples are given: *"progressive acquisition of maternal role behaviors related to seeking and gaining experience in child care"* and *"beginning maternal acquaintance related to early contact with newborn"* (p. 14).

Stevens (1988) also proposes use of both problem and wellness nursing diagnoses for postpartum maternity clients. She suggests using a combination NANDA system and a systems/adaptation conceptual framework. The psychosocial systems she presents for assessment include parenting, home maintenance management, family process and coping, diversional activities, social interaction, and self-concept. Examples of wellness nursing diagnoses include *"progress in parenting tasks"*; *"progressive family coping after delivery"*; and *"progressive self-concept, mothering role performance"* (pp. 332–333).

Starn and Niederhauser (1990) present an MCN developmental/diagnostic model based on developmental concepts that combines problem-oriented and wellness-oriented nursing diagnoses for childbearing/childrearing families. Cognitive and moral development as well as psychosocial and physiological concepts are included in the model. Examples of adaptive nursing diagnoses are *"efficient developmental progression related to appropriate stimulation"* and *"appropriate health maintenance related to proper preventive practices"* (p. 181). There could be confusion as to whether these statements are diagnoses or client goals. In either instance, the desired response is already present and little remains for the nurse to do to help the client achieve a healthy state.

Henrikson, Wall, Lethbridge, and McClurg (1992) agree that maternity nurses have had difficulty using problem-oriented nursing diagnoses with clients who are essentially well. Believing that the nursing diagnosis is a means by which the profession communicates independent practice, they suggest the maternity nurses can no longer ignore their use. As a result of their beliefs, they developed the nursing diagnosis *"effective breastfeeding"* and present a standardized nursing care plan for clients with that diagnosis.

~ Wellness Diagnoses and Functional Health Patterns

One of the most extensive groups of wellness diagnoses was developed by Houldin, Saltstein, and Ganley (1987). The authors organize these wellness-oriented diagnoses according to functional health patterns and build upon utilization of client strengths as the basis of their diagnoses. Additionally, they maintain that these diagnoses demand a focus on wellness rather than the usual illness orientation. Use of these diagnoses facilitates development of strengths, which help the client achieve higher and higher levels of wellness. Examples include *"potential for achieving satisfactory hydration status to meet metabolic needs"* (p. 75); *"self care, independence"* (p. 97); and *"spiritual strength"* (p. 141).

SUMMARY

Although controversy still exists about the place for wellness diagnoses in nursing, interest in this topic is increasing. A growing body of literature describes the use of wellness nursing diagnoses in various clinical settings. No one particular approach to writing wellness diagnoses exists as reflected in this literature review. Articles in the literature suggest various ways to write such diagnoses ranging from very detailed descriptions of client responses to diagnostic judgment statements, at a more conceptual level, which reflect a client's response to a healthy condition. Perhaps this fluidity is necessary as the concept of wellness diagnoses evolves. Nevertheless, conceptual difficulties do exist with some of the proposed methods of writing wellness diagnoses. Some diagnoses sound like goals, others describe specific behaviors and leave one wondering on what basis the nurse can plan care, and others are so long they are impractical and unwieldy. However, as nurses work with these diagnoses, refinement will occur and new diagnoses will be presented. The progression of these ideas is exciting and can only benefit the client who does not have an illness, but needs guidance in working through a developmental or maturational task or seeks assistance in health promotion.

References

Allen, C.J. (1989). Incorporating a wellness perspective for nursing diagnosis in practice. In R.M. Carroll-Johnson (ed.), *Classification of Nursing Diagnoses: Proceedings of the Eighth Conference North American Nursing Diagnosis Association* (pp. 37–42). Philadelphia: Lippincott.

Bestard, S., and Courteney, M. (1990). Focusing on wellness. *The Canadian Nurse*, 86(11), 24–25.

Flagler, S., and Nicoll, L. (1990). A framework for the psychological aspects of pregnancy. *NAACOG's Clinical Issues in Perinatal and Women's Health Nursing*, 1(3), 267–278.

Frenn, M.D., Jacobs, C.A., Lee, H.A., Sanger, M.T., and Strong, K.A. (1987). Delphi survey to gain consensus on wellness and health promotion nursing diagnoses. In A.M. McLane (ed.), *Classification of Nursing Diagnoses: Proceedings of the Seventh Conference North American Nursing Diagnosis Association* (pp. 154–159). St. Louis: Mosby.

Gleit, C.J., and Tatro, S. (1981). Nursing diagnoses for healthy individuals. *Nursing and Health Care*, 11(8), 456–457.

Gordon, M. (1994). *Nursing Diagnosis: Process and Application*, 3rd ed. St. Louis: Mosby.

Guzzetta, C.E., Bunton, S.D., Prinkey, L.A., Sherer, A.P., and Seifert, P.C. (1988). Unitary person assessment tool: Easing problems with nursing diagnoses. *Focus on Critical Care*, 15(2), 12–24.

Henrikson, M., Wall, G., Lethbridge, D., and McClurg, V. (1992). Nursing diagnosis and obstetric, gynecologic, and neonatal nursing: Breastfeeding as an example. *JOGNN*, 21, 446–456.

Hornberger, C.A. (1989). Perceived stressors, perceived stress response, and level of cardiac reactivity in a wellness sample. Unpublished master's thesis: University of Kansas.

Houldin, A.D., Saltstein, S.W., and Ganley, K.M. (1987). *Nursing Diagnoses for Wellness*. Philadelphia: Lippincott

Keeling, A.W. (1988). Health promotion in coronary care and step-down units: Focus on the family—linking research to practice. *Heart and Lung*, 17, 28–34.

Lee, H.A., and Frenn, M.D. (1987). The use of nursing diagnoses for health promotion in community practice. *Nursing Clinics of North America*, 22, 981–987.

Lyons, J.F., and Hester, N.O. (1987). Research-generated nursing diagnoses for healthy school-age children. *Issues in Comprehensive Pediatric Nursing*, 10, 149–159.

Martens, K. (1986). Let's diagnose strengths, not just problems. *American Journal of Nursing*, 86, 192–193.

Mundinger, M.O., and Jauron, G.D. (1975). Developing a nursing diagnosis. *Nursing Outlook*, 23(2), 94–98.

Neufeld, A., and Harrison, M.J. (1994). Analysis of nursing diagnoses for population groups in the community. In R.M. Carroll-Johnson and M. Paquette (eds.), *Classification of Nursing Diagnoses: Proceedings of the Tenth Conference North American Nursing Diagnosis Association* (pp. 239–241). Philadelphia: Lippincott.

Nicoletti, A. (1991). Specialty organizations: Nursing diagnoses use and issues—A panel presentation (Nurses Association of the American College of Obstetrics and Gynecology). In R. M. Carroll-Johnson (ed.), *Classification of Nursing Diagnoses: Proceedings of the Ninth Conference North American Nursing Diagnosis Association* (pp. 215–217). Philadelphia: Lippincott.

Popkess, S.A. (1981). Diagnosing your patient's strengths. *Nursing*, 11(7), 34–39.

Popkess-Vawter, S. (1984). Strength-oriented nursing diagnoses. In M.J. Kim, G.K. McFarland, and A.M. McLane (eds.), *Classification of Nursing Diagnoses: Proceedings of the Fifth National Conference North American Nursing Diagnosis Association* (pp. 443–440). St. Louis: Mosby.

Popkess-Vawter, S. (1991). Wellness nursing diagnoses: To be or not to be? *Nursing Diagnosis*, 2(1), 19–25.

Popkess. S., and Pinnell, N. (1987). Yes: Accentuate the positive. *American Journal of Nursing*, 87, 1211, 1216.

Ridenour, N. (1994). Aggregate nursing diagnoses for community health. In R.M. Carroll-Johnson and M. Paquette (eds.), *Classification of Nursing Diagnoses: Proceedings of the Tenth Conference North American Nursing Diagnosis Association* (pp. 149–153). Philadelphia: Lippincott.

Roy, Sr., C., and Andrews, H.A. (1991). *The Roy Adaptation Model*. Norwalk: Appleton & Lange.

Standards of Clinical Nursing Practice (1991). Washington, DC: American Nurses Association.

Starn, J., and Niederhauser, V. (1990). An MCN model for nursing diagnosis to focus intervention. *MCN: The American Journal of Maternal-Child Nursing*, 15, 180–183.

Stevens, K. (1988). Nursing diagnoses in wellness childbearing settings. *JOGNN*, 17, 329–336.

Stolte, K. (1986a). A complementary view of nursing diagnosis. *Public Health Nursing*, 3(1), 23–28.

Stolte, K.M. (1986b). Nursing diagnosis and the childbearing woman. *MCN: The American Journal of Maternal-Child Nursing*, 11, 13–15.

Stolte, K. (1989). Using health-oriented nursing diagnoses in medical-surgical nursing. *Journal of Advanced Medical-Surgical Nursing, 1*, 73–82.

Tatro, S., and Gleit, C.J. (1983). A wellness model for nursing: Promoting high level wellness in any setting through independent nursing functions. *Nursing Leadership, 6*(1), 5–9.

Taylor-Loughran, A.E. (1990). Toward a nursing diagnosis definition. *Clinical Nurse Specialist, 4*, 71–75.

Zetelmaier, M.A. (1983). Nursing assessment and diagnosis (Letter to the editor). *JOGN Nursing, 12*, 219.

18
~

Selected Annotated Bibliography

~ Wellness Nursing Diagnoses

A small, but growing, body of literature is available related to development and use of wellness nursing diagnoses. For those who wish to read further in the field, a selected group of articles and book chapters is presented here with annotations.

~ Articles

Bestard, S., and Courteney, M. (1990). Focusing on wellness. *The Canadian Nurse*, 86(11), 24–25.

 The authors maintain that promoting wellness is an important aspect of nursing care and use the nursing process to demonstrate how wellness nursing diagnoses can be developed. A case study is presented.

Gleit, C.J., and Tatro, S. (1981). Nursing diagnoses for healthy individuals. *Nursing and Health Care*, 11, 456–457.

 This is an early article that focuses on including wellness components in a nursing diagnosis. The authors assert that nurses must build on client strengths. Using high-level wellness as a framework, they propose that primary prevention needs to be incorporated into the definition of nursing diagnosis.

Keeling, A.W. (1988). Health promotion in coronary care and stepdown units: Focus on the family—linking research to practice. *Heart and Lung*, 17, 28–34.

Discussion of a study that evaluated an assessment tool to gather data from wives of patients with acute myocardial infarction and used the data to formulate nursing diagnoses and interventions for this group of clients. Both illness-oriented and wellness-oriented nursing diagnoses are presented.

Lee, H.A., and Frenn, M.D. (1987). The use of nursing diagnoses for health promotion in community practice. *Nursing Clinics of North America, 22*, 981–987.

Although community health nurses use both positive and problem-focused nursing diagnoses in practice, these authors maintain that positive diagnoses reflect a health promotion orientation more accurately than diagnoses that examine patient vulnerability and deal with potential problems. They assert that a holistic database must contain information about client strengths. Case studies are presented and selected health promotion nursing diagnoses are included that were obtained from a pilot study of community health nurses.

Lyons, J.F., and Hester, N.O. (1987). Research-generated nursing diagnoses for healthy school-age children. *Issues in Comprehensive Pediatric Nursing, 10*, 149–159.

These authors present a case for positive nursing diagnoses in pediatric primary health care settings. They believe these diagnoses would help ensure that complete assessments are made as well as increase professional accountability. A system linking health category, nursing diagnosis, and indicators of the diagnosis is presented, including 12 categories with a total of 22 wellness-oriented nursing diagnoses for school-age children.

Martens, K. (1986). Let's diagnose strengths, not just problems. *American Journal of Nursing, 86*, 192–193.

Believing that the nurse is concerned with helping clients maintain health, this author emphasizes the importance of identifying and documenting client strengths. The nurse can then build on these strengths to prevent or overcome problems. A case study is presented, a strength diagnosis is defined, and examples of diagnostic statements are proposed.

Popkess, S.A. (1981). Diagnosing your patient's strengths. *Nursing, 11*(7), 34–39.

An early proponent of wellness diagnoses, this author describes identification of both client problems and strengths as a nursing responsibility. A nursing assessment format is included to demonstrate ways to diagnose strengths.

Popkess-Vawter, S. (1991). Wellness nursing diagnoses: To be or not to be? *Nursing Diagnosis, 2*(1), 19–25.

By reviewing the literature, the author describes the evolution of thought about wellness nursing diagnoses in NANDA. She presents both pros and cons related to the issue; however, she emphasizes her position that wellness nursing diagnoses are appropriate for all types of clients across the scope of nursing practice. In particular, she believes wellness diagnoses are useful if wellness behaviors are not fully established or supports are not adequate to maintain wellness behaviors. Examples of wellness diagnoses are given for each clinical area.

Popkess-Vawter, S., and Pinnell, N. (1987). Yes: Accentuate the positive. *American Journal of Nursing, 87,* 1211, 1216.

Members of the Mid-America Regional Nursing Diagnosis Conference Group assert that health concerns and practices must be incorporated into client assessment for holistic care. If health-oriented nursing diagnoses are used, assessment of wellness programs can be done. Additionally, the authors assert that patient independence and satisfaction can be increased.

Starn, J., and Niederhauser, V. (1990). An MCN model for nursing diagnosis to focus intervention. *MCN: The American Journal of Maternal-Child Nursing, 15,* 180–183.

The authors of this article have developed an MCN developmental/diagnostic model to deal with nursing diagnoses for child-rearing and childbearing families. This model is based on developmental concepts and includes both problem-oriented and health-oriented diagnoses. Case studies for childbearing and child-rearing situations are presented.

Stevens, K.A. (1988). Nursing diagnosis in wellness childbearing settings. *JOGNN, 17,* 329–336.

This author explains that substituting a positive word for the negative one in the NANDA classification system would be one way to include health-oriented nursing diagnoses in wellness childbearing settings. Combining this approach with use of a systems/adaptation conceptual framework would facilitate development of diagnoses for the well postpartum client. A table including transition from negative NANDA diagnoses to positive wellness diagnoses is presented.

Stolte, K.M. (1986). Nursing diagnosis and the childbearing woman. *MCN: The American Journal of Maternal-Child Nursing, 11*(1), 13–15.

It has been difficult to use the NANDA diagnosis list in maternity nursing since most maternity clients are healthy women. The author advocates the use of positive nursing diagnoses and includes several examples of diagnoses with goal statements and nursing interventions.

Stolte, K. (1986). A complementary view of nursing diagnosis. *Public Health Nursing, 3*(1), 23–28.

This article describes how to write positive nursing diagnoses and gives examples of their use in community health nursing.

Stolte, K. (1989). Using health-oriented nursing diagnoses in medical-surgical nursing. *Journal of Advanced Medical-Surgical Nursing, 1,* 73–82.

An overview of the development and use of health-oriented nursing diagnoses is presented. Examples of this type of diagnosis for critical care and acute medical-surgical nursing clients are given.

Tatro, S., and Gleit, C.J. (1983). A wellness model for nursing: Promoting high level wellness in any setting through independent nursing functions. *Nursing Leadership, 6*(1), 5–9.

Using a wellness model, these authors assert that nursing includes strength building. They refine nursing diagnosis to include healthy as well as unhealthy responses. Case studies are included and wellness diagnoses are provided.

~ *Books/Book Chapters*

Allen, C.J. (1989). Incorporating a wellness perspective for nursing diagnosis in practice. In R.M. Carroll-Johnson (ed.), *Classification of Nursing Diagnoses: Proceedings of the Eighth Conference North American Nursing Diagnosis Association* (pp. 37–42). Philadelphia: Lippincott.

An overview of the use of nursing diagnoses by public health nurses, and the problems associated with their use, revealed that the lack of a focus on wellness, health promotion, and disease prevention is a major concern. Several solutions to address this concern include use of the Omaha taxonomy, modification of NANDA diagnoses to include positive modifiers, and generation of new diagnoses. Examples of wellness diagnoses are given.

Frenn, M.D., Jacobs, C.A., Lee, H.A., Sanger, M.T., and Strong, K.A. (1987). Delphi survey to gain consensus on wellness and health promotion nursing diagnoses. In A.M. McLane (ed.), *Classification of Nursing Diagnoses: Proceedings of the Seventh Conference North American Nursing Diagnosis Association* (pp. 154–159). St. Louis: Mosby.

Using the Delphi technique, the authors conducted a study that generated wellness and health promotion nursing diagnoses. The diagnoses are listed and reasons for using them are also given.

Henrikson, M.L., Wall, G., Lethbridge, D., and McClurg, V.E. (1991). Effective breastfeeding. In R.M. Carroll-Johnson (ed.), *Classification of Nursing Diagnoses: Proceedings of the Ninth Conference North American Nursing Diagnosis Association* (pp. 352–357). Philadelphia: Lippincott.

As a part of a bigger study on validation of nursing diagnoses, this particular diagnosis was considered. Defining characteristics and related factors are presented. Future plans for additional diagnoses related to breastfeeding are described.

Houldin A.D., Saltstein, S.W., and Ganley, K.M. (1987). *Nursing Diagnoses for Wellness.* Philadelphia: Lippincott.

This handbook presents a taxonomy of wellness nursing diagnoses based on functional health patterns. Examples of these diagnoses are given along with contributing factors and defining characteristics.

Nicoletti, A. (1989). Nurses Association of the American College of Obstetrics and Gynecology. In R.M. Carroll-Johnson (ed.), *Classification of Nursing Diagnosis: Proceedings of the Eighth Conference North American Nursing Diagnosis Association* (pp. 215–217). Philadelphia: Lippincott.

As a representative from NAACOG to the NANDA meeting, the author describes the frustration maternity nurses have in trying to use problem-oriented nursing diagnoses with well clients. Issues related to patient education diagnoses as well as physiologic diagnoses are described.

Pender, N.J. (1989). Languaging a health perspective for NANDA taxonomy on research and theory. In R.M. Carroll-Johnson (ed.), *Classification of Nursing Diagnosis: Proceedings of the Eighth Conference North American Nursing Diagnosis Association* (pp. 31–36). Philadelphia: Lippincott.

The author suggests that two parallel, complementary taxonomies for nursing diagnoses could be developed. One would relate to potential or actual health problems; the other would relate to human strengths and resources. A second approach would be to combine the two for a taxonomy of human health/illness responses. Either method would include health promotion which, up to the present, has been limited in approaches to nursing diagnosis.

Popkess-Vawter, S. (1984). Strength-oriented nursing diagnoses. In M.J. Kim, G.K. McFarland, and A.M. McLane (eds.), *Classification of Nursing Diagnoses: Proceedings of the Fifth National Conference North American Nursing Diagnosis Association* (pp. 433–440). St. Louis: Mosby.

One of the earliest articles on positive nursing diagnoses, it posits the value of strength-oriented diagnoses and presents a list of positive nursing diagnoses as well as sources that will provide data for these diagnoses.

Stolte, K. (1994). Health-oriented nursing diagnoses: Development and use. In R.M. Carroll-Johnson and M. Paquette (eds.), *Classification of Nursing Diagnoses: Proceedings of the Tenth Conference North American Nursing Diagnosis Association* (pp. 143–148). Philadelphia: Lippincott.

The author discusses the value of health-oriented nursing diagnoses and proposes a format for writing such diagnoses. Examples are given. The material in the article is amplified in the first three chapters of this book.

Tripp, S., and Stachowiak, B. (1989). Nursing diagnosis: Health seeking behaviors (specify). In R.M. Carroll-Johnson (ed.), *Classification of Nursing Diagnoses: Proceedings of the Eighth Conference North American Nursing Diagnosis Association* (pp. 433–436). Philadelphia: Lippincott.

The article introduces a new nursing diagnosis appropriate for clients who actively seek to improve their presently healthy state. Defining characteristics and supportive materials are included.

Warren, J.J. (1991). Implications of introducing axes into a classification system. In R.M. Carroll-Johnson (ed.), *Classification of Nursing Diagnoses: Proceedings of the Ninth Conference North American Nursing Diagnosis Association* (pp. 38–43). Philadelphia: Lippincott.

The possibility of introducing axes into the NANDA classification is discussed. Four axes are proposed: unit of analysis (individual, family, or community), age group, wellness, and illness. Implications of these axes for taxonomists, researchers, administrators, and practitioners are reviewed.

Appendix
~

Wellness Nursing Diagnoses Listed by Chapter

Chapter 3: Assessment of Client Strengths

Increasing knowledge about adequate nutrition

Improving nutritional intake

Compliance with prescribed diet

Increasing ability to avoid stressful situations

Beginning practice of stress management techniques

Increasing ability to maintain stress reduction through consistent use of stress management techniques

Developing goals for physical exercise

Beginning maintenance of exercise regimen

Beginning acceptance of responsibility for self-care

Accepting responsibility for self-care

Progressive identification and elimination of negative health care practices

Initiating a program of stress reduction

Actively seeking knowledge about medical treatment or disease process

Beginning preparation for maturational/developmental event (specify)

Anticipating lifestyle changes required for maturational/ developmental event

Learning new skills required for adaption to developmental/ maturational event

Planning for new role

Pride in ability to master new role
Progressive attainment of role behaviors
Progressive interaction with support group members
Recognizing interdependence among family members
Seeking interaction with others to learn new skill/role
Progressive religious faith
Maintaining strong spiritual foundation
Maintaining hope and trust in higher power
Progressive ability to forgive self and/or others
Continued belief in meaning and purpose of life
At peace with self and/or health status
Increasing desire to improve health status
Increasing ability to evaluate strengths and weaknesses in order to
  set realistic self-care goals
Feelings of satisfaction with past achievements
Increasing self-confidence
Beginning skill in use of medical equipment/technology (specify)
Modifying home environment to accommodate medical
  technology
Increasing compliance with prescribed treatment
Motivation to follow prescribed medical treatment
Ongoing use of coping skills
Demonstrated ability to cope with stress

Chapter 4: Wellness Nursing Diagnoses for the Childbearing Family

Beginning acceptance of reality of the pregnancy
Seeking early prenatal care
Increasing joy about being pregnant
Progressive incorporation of physical changes of pregnancy into
  lifestyle
Progressive acceptance of reality of the fetus
Beginning preparation of environment (nesting) for new infant
Beginning prenatal attachment
Examining relationship with own mother
Developing a working relationship directed toward mutual support
  during pregnancy and parenting
Recognizing family interdependence
Beginning fantasies about the infant's personality

Beginning maternal–infant attachment
Resolving conflict between fantasized infant and actual infant
Beginning attainment of mothering role
Integrating fantasy role with actual mothering role
Progressive preparation for labor
Creating a labor plan to communicate personal desires for labor
    experience
Maintaining control during labor
Acquiring role of labor coach
Beginning establishment of breastfeeding
Increasing confidence in infant care skills
Beginning integration of the infant into the family
Beginning adjustment to multiple roles
Adequate oxygen exchange
Maintenance of thermoregulation
Adequate nutritional intake
Progressive transition to extrauterine life
Progressive synchrony with mother
Beginning to elicit caretaking behaviors
Progressive self-comforting behavior

Chapter 5: Wellness Nursing Diagnoses for Infants

Progressive development of motor skills
Beginning sense of trust
Beginning recognition of event sequencing
Performance of imitative acts
Beginning recognition of object permanence
Beginning acquisition of verbal skills
Progressive interaction with family members
Beginning expression of pleasure associated with repetitive
    activities

Chapter 6: Wellness Nursing Diagnoses for Toddlers and Preschool Children

Progressive refining of motor skills
Beginning sense of autonomy
Beginning sense of initiative

Rapid increase in language skills
Preoperational thinking
Beginning social interaction through imitation
Increasing self-expression in play activities

Chapter 7: Wellness Nursing Diagnoses for School-Age Children

Continuing refinement of motor skills
Beginning sense of industry
Beginning recognition of personal competence
Eagerness to engage in social activities
Joy and satisfaction with personal accomplishments
Increasing ability for complex thinking
Successful achievement in school
Increasing ability to consider alternative viewpoints
Beginning cooperative play
Increasing social interaction
Beginning adaption to new school
Incorporating new family members into personal social system
Beginning adaptation to chronic illness
Conquering fears of hospitalization
Incorporating physical changes into lifestyle

Chapter 8: Wellness Nursing Diagnoses for Adolescents

Beginning sense of personal identity
Increasing interest in opposite sex
Incorporating secondary sex changes into body image
Beginning formulation of occupational goals
Beginning separation from family authority
Increasing consideration of others' opinions
Increasing ability for abstract reasoning
Developing potentially long-lasting relationships
Developing relationships with opposite-sex peers
Increasing personal interests and hobbies

Chapter 9: Wellness Nursing Diagnoses for Adults: Early Adulthood

Increasing separation from family authority
Beginning adult identity
Assuming leadership role in community
Beginning balance of personal and work responsibilities
Developing relationships within the work force
Increasing problem-solving ability
Defining marital role behaviors
Beginning acceptance of parenting role
Reevaluating and developing parenting skills consistent with needs
    of growing children
Adjusting to career change
Adjusting to relocation
Balancing multiple roles
Developing long-term goals for family security

Chapter 10: Wellness Nursing Diagnoses for Adults: Middle Adulthood

Pride in accomplishments
Adapting to the growing family
Adjusting to changes in family configuration
Adapting to minor health changes
Reevaluating personal goals
Increasing acceptance of self
Adapting to increased financial responsibilities
Exploring alternatives for parental care
Planning for retirement

Chapter 11: Wellness Nursing Diagnoses for Adults: Late Adulthood

Adapting to retirement
Reestablishing spousal relationships
Progressive adjustment to physiological changes
Assuming responsibility for own health
Participating in satisfying activities
Developing a pattern for daily living

Involvement in service activities
Satisfaction with past and present life as lived
Increasing recognition of one's own strengths

Chapter 12: Wellness Nursing Diagnoses for Adults in Critical Care

Maintaining consciousness and cognitive function
Maintaining effective communication
Progressing through the grieving process
Maintaining muscle strength
Complying with the treatment plan
Facilitating own emotional balance
Acquiring knowledge
Questioning care
Improving activity tolerance
Retaining sense of control
Maintaining social support networks
Maintaining family cohesiveness
Maintaining consistent self-concept
Accepting limitations from illness/injury
Maintaining sensory input balance
Obtaining normal sensory input
Maintaining usual sleep/rest cycle
Progressive healing of myocardium
Maintaining normal blood pressure during position changes
Effective airway clearance
Maintaining normal skin integrity
Progessive weaning from ventilator
Sustained ability to carry out self-care activities
Progressing toward fluid and electrolyte balance
Progressing toward nutritional balance

Chapter 13: Wellness Nursing Diagnoses in Home Health Care

Client

Maintaining current mobility
Progressive restoration of previous mobility status

Actively seeking knowledge about medical treatment or disease
    process
Increasing acceptance of responsibility for self-care
Increasing compliance with prescribed treatment
Increasing utilization of community resources
Increasing knowledge about adequate nutrition
Compliance with prescribed diet
Increasing social interaction while eating
Knowledge about prescribed fluid needs
Increasing knowledge about medication needs specific to fluid and
    electrolytes
Progressive social interaction
Actively seeking resources to meet spiritual needs
Beginning acceptance of role change
Creating a safe environment conducive to health care
Beginning transition to home care
Beginning skill in use of medical equipment/technology (specify)

Caregiver

Mobilizing efforts to meet personal/family needs
Beginning adjustment to caregiving status
Planning flexible routine for caregiving

Chapter 14: Wellness Nursing Diagnoses
for Groups

Continued consistency of group norms
Progressive group interdependence
Increasingly supportive group climate

Chapter 15: Wellness Nursing Diagnoses
for Families

Progressive development of mutually satisfying relationship
Beginning development of the family unit
Developing ties to extended family
Increasing allocation by couple of time alone without the infant
Progressive development of family child care patterns
Increasing social interaction appropriate for children's ages and
    abilities

Progressive inclusion of children in family discussions and decisions

Adapting individual roles within the family to accommodate changes in family configuration or size

Increasing utilization of family and community resources

Increasing ability of individual family members to give and take in order to meet each other's needs

Reevaluating and developing parenting skills consistent with needs of growing children (see Chapter 9)

Maintaining balance between independent and dependent needs of children

Continued commitment to family values

Integration of new family member

Beginning reestablishment of a mutually satisfying couple relationship

Progressive reestablishment of a mutually satisfying couple relationship

Progressive participation in satisfying service activities

Maintenance of intergenerational relationships

Satisfaction with family life as lived

Progressive adaptation to changes in family lifestyle occurring from loss

Chapter 16: Wellness Nursing Diagnoses for Communities

Progressive community interaction for problem solving and goal identification

Progressive participation in community goal-directed activities

Index